On a Knife's Edge

A Young Girl's Journey through Borderline Personality Disorder

Michelle Karpus

chipmunkapublishing

the mental health publisher

Michelle Karpus

All rights reserved, no part of this publication may be reproduced by any means, electronic, mechanical photocopying, documentary, film or in any other format without prior written permission of the publisher.

Published by

Chipmunkapublishing

PO Box 6872

Brentwood

Essex CM13 1ZT

United Kingdom

http://www.chipmunkapublishing.com

Copyright © Michelle Karpus 2010

Chipmunkapublishing gratefully acknowledge the support of Arts Council England.

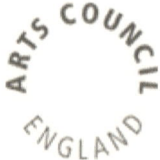

On a Knife's Edge

Prologue

Waking up to the sound of a large bird squawking outside my window, I picked up my cuddly toy Posey and trotted down the stairs. Usually on my way I would go and wake up my baby sister by nuzzling her on the head with teddy, but today she was not in her cot. The muffled smell of damp and dust surrounded me as I half walked and half crawled around searching for the baby. There was a soft muffled cry from downstairs, and a tiny wave of panic struck my tiny five year old body. I lay on my tummy and rolled down the stairs, bumping and bumping until I hit the bottom. As usual, my mother was sitting down on the sofa crying softly to herself, and any amount of begging for her to stop would not be welcomed. My baby sister was in her arms, fast asleep. I wanted to get to my sister to keep her safe; this was my new aim in life. I did not want the mother to hold her; I did not know what she would do.

Perhaps I could pretend this was a game. It was still early and my grandmother would not be there for a long time, at least ten minutes. I set up my dolls house and put little tea cups and dollies in a circle. They seemed to be laughing at me, mocking my pathetic rescue attempts, but I could not be stopped. Surely my mother would understand that I needed my sister to complete this circle. I took my sister gently from my mother's arms, and sat her down. My sister opened her mouth and let out a tenacious yell that rung in my ears. My mother cried harder, and my sister screamed louder, and I felt like it was a competition and I was the referee. I had hidden all the knives in the doll's house, so nothing bad could happen. My mother was searching for these knives, and when they were not to be found she grabbed a pair of scissors. She rolled up her sleeves and I knew what was coming. I snatched them out of her fingers with all the power and force of a twelve year old, and threw them across the room. My mother sat back down on the sofa and cried again, running her fingers through her unwashed hair. I took my sister into the kitchen; it was time to make breakfast.

Weetabix with milk was our favourite, so that is what we had. Milk was spilt and the Weetabix was swimming in a brown mushy mess, but it was all I could manage with my undeveloped fingers. My sister was laughing now, making a gurgling sound as I stuck my tongue out and hid behind my hands. With the monotone baby laugh I tried to block out the thought of my mother back in the other room, but each second bought a new sense of anticipation. My breath quickened as I prepared myself to protect my sister, and where was my grandmother? Wasn't she normally here by now? I formed a plan in my head. I could push my sister in my dolly's pushchair, and we could go up the hill and take the red and yellow bus to our Grandmother's house.

The silence in the other room was torture for me; I would have preferred the blissful sound of sobbing instead of the fear of the unknown. I knew something bad was happening, something very bad. Then my mother burst in. Blood was dripping from her arm; she must have found the knives. She waved this bloody mess in my face whilst screaming, look what you made me do, you selfish little brat. I covered my ears and tried to sink in the ground, pushing my hands onto my ears as hard as they would go but I could still hear her. I screamed to myself, just to make sure I was still there. I carried on until my mother scooped me up in her arms and rocked me gently, making soothing noises. She was back, for a moment she was back again. I snuggled my face into her neck, and wrapped my arms around her.

On a Knife's Edge

She was back again, and everything was going to be ok, everything was going to be ok, everything was going to be ok.

Michelle Karpus

On a Knife's Edge

Chapter 1

Everyone struggles to fit in. Everyone tries to be unique. Everyone strives to find that balance.

Julie was never as alone as when she was surrounded by all these people in the large room. From childhood they all thought she was different. She did not join in much with the other children; no, Julie was the one at the back of her classroom, fingers in her mouth and crying. What she was crying for, she did not know. She hated being in nursery, yet she hated being at home. She was not crying for her mother who was at home sobbing a lot of the time. Her baby sister was there, but already Julie did not like her. Since her arrival her mother had not been the same, depressed all the time. The new baby was supposed to be exciting, but all it bought was sadness.

The familiar grey haired lady came in with a tremendous gift; it had blue shiny paper on it, and a big gold ribbon. Julie fought to rip open the bow, her small fingers hurting with the effort. The grey haired lady came back with a pair of scissors, and Julie found herself panting with excitement. She pulled at the paper, tearing big chunks out and a large pink box was showing itself more and more. It was a doll, a pretty doll with long, blonde hair just like Julie's. She was so pleased with it, but she sat quietly and stared. How to show she was pleased? She did not know, but she knew she wanted to open the box, but it looked so nice like that.
"Here, let Grandma help you," the grey haired woman said. She opened the box and lifted the doll for Julie to hold.
"I have my baby, just like mummy," Julie had wanted

to say, but instead she muttered, "baby, mummy." Grandma understood.

Then mummy came in, holding a small parcel of blankets. "Oh, don't give her any more dolls. She ruins them. She draws on them, cuts their hair, and pulls off their legs. I just can't be bothered to waste my money on them."

"Well, you didn't waste your money, I did," said Grandma.

Julie listened to her mummy's wailing voice in the background, knowing it would not be long before she was crying. Crying again. Julie wants it to stop, and then she feels it. The warm rush of feeling surrounded her from the waist down. It was warm and wet and cosy, but then it began to grow cold. Very cold and uncomfortable. That is when mummy put her back in nappies.

The big white keys were amazing. They had little black keys above them, and when Julie touched one it made a noise. Each key made a different noise; each black key was even more fun. But what was this man saying to her; making her play the ones she did not want to play. No, that was not right. That was not the key she wanted to play. She wanted to go up and low, not in the middle. Why was he grabbing her finger and making her play the ones she did not want to play? This was not right; this was not what she saw in her head. She covered her ears and screamed, until she felt someone lifting her, and smacking her hard across her bottom until she stopped. She did not want to see those black and white keys anymore.

Sitting in that doctor's waiting room and waiting. What was she waiting for? Her friend Anna sat besides her holding her hand, offering the occasional everything will be OK smile. The doctor was over seven foot tall, long black beard, hunched over to avoid hitting his head. He grinned and moved his arms in direction of the door. She picked up her coat and shakily followed him through the long blue corridor, up the blank white stairs and into a little room, Anna trailing at her feet. For the first time in hours she actually felt pretty calm, if only for a moment. She knew something was going to happen. At last something was going to be done; she was going to get the help she so desperately needed. She knew for certain that she needed someone to help her, or she would surely die. She would die and never be able to see her friends, never hear the sounds of children's laughter as they played on the swings, never watch a flock of birds in the sky. It was really a very basic choice; live or die. Which would it be?

When your heart is crying it is very hard for anyone to hear because it is hidden deep within your chest. When you are crying out in pain it is camouflaged within your dry tears that refuse to spill. Instead you soak up the pain like a sponge, but sooner or later a sponge has to burst. There is only so much water it can hold. There is only so much pain one can bear.

The first time she had come into hospital to treat her cuts had been years ago. A past life time with a totally different friend. This friend was dead now. Long gone and never to be seen again except in her dreams. Julie quietly remembered these dreams and felt a warm feeling, then quickly followed by a stabbing ache in her heart at the lost memories. Anna was here now, and Anna was going to help her. She was going to be her friend and she was going to push for her to be helped. Julie remembered a little baby bird she had once found with a broken wing. Julie scooped up the bird and took it home. It turned out the wing was not broken, because a few hours later it got up and flew to the top of the cupboard. Her mother phoned the RSPCA who explained that the bird was probably tired and wanted a rest. The wing was not really broken after all. Julie was mistaken. She envied that bird.

Her experience in that first time she had gone to hospital for stitches the nurse had been kind. She had been non-judgemental and she had cared. If only all the nurses could be like that. If only Julie would be forever met with the patience and understanding of this nurse. "We need to get you some help," she said. Julie had been asking for help. She had been going to her psychiatrist and asking for help and she had been promised help. It was on the way. There was an eighteen month waiting list for a psychologist; sometimes it went up to two years. She had been referred, but she had nothing. She was left. Just like baby P, Elliott had remarked.

"How do you feel today?" the doctor asked.
I want to die. "Fine." That was a lie. That was an obvious lie, but how can you tell the truth? How can you say what is really on your mind? I need someone to help me. I need someone to hold me close and tell me everything is going to be ok, to comfort me like a baby. To soothe me and let me know they care, but the arms are empty. There is nothing. Please save me please will someone not help me? Well at least Anna cared. She cared enough to fight for her. To fight for help, when all the fight left in Julie had gone. All the strength had disappeared and she was left defeated.
"Julie, Julie, can you hear me?" Dr Nicolas was asking, "Julie, do you think you need to go to hospital? Shall we see what happens for one more night? Reassess you tomorrow and then decide whether to put you in hospital?" Julie nodded. The calm moment had passed. Now she didn't care. She did not want to be

alive anymore. She just could not cope and she was fairly certain by now that nobody was going to help her. She had been promised so much help and support for so long, with no results. She was supposed to have CBT, but was told that she was too severe. She was supposed to go to therapy groups, but as her sister attended them she could not go. She was becoming accustomed to not being helped. Death was the only way out. Perhaps tonight she would succeed, or perhaps tonight she would not feel like dying. Maybe the voices in the walls would stop bullying her and pressurising her to die, and maybe she would feel peace and tranquillity. She did not know, she did not care. But Anna would not let her give up, would not wait one more night. She stood up and made herself heard.

"I am not taking her home," she screeched, "if I take her home she is going to KILL HERSELF. I am NOT taking her home for one more night. You don't understand. Last night she took an overdose, the night before she tried to strangle herself. I am NOT taking her home."

Keith pulled Anna out into the hallway and spoke to her. Julie stayed in the waiting room on her own. With Anna gone, she felt so isolated, if only for a short moment. The overwhelming urge to die seized upon her, took over her body. She was lucky she would not have to go to hospital as it meant she really could kill herself. She longed for the sweet release of death. The finality when she could be at peace and be with her best friend Emma. The pain was all too much and it never seemed to subside. She wanted to die so badly just to find tranquillity. Life had no purpose. Life was a cruel place. Death was the only way out. The voices in the walls dug deep into her ears and settled in the pit of her stomach. Die you must die they chanted. She went into a corner and took her handbag. She wrapped it round her neck and twisted it round tighter and tighter until she could not breathe. She felt her pain leave her body and start to float away, but then suddenly Anna was there unwrapping the bag. "See! I won't take her home like this. I can't be with her twenty four hours, I can't. Please please help her!"

Keith agreed. She could not go home. He agreed to find her a bed. She was going to be admitted into hospital tonight. She was going to get some help, or so they thought. Julie started to resist the idea of going into hospital, only to be told that she had two choices; either she go into hospital voluntarily, or they would make her.

"I'm not convinced hospital is the best place for her," Dr Nathaniel had said for the past few months. "It will not change anything. She will still harm herself. She will still be depressed, but she would have some silly foreign nurse telling her what to do. She will not do well in hospital with this diagnosis." Julie was terrified at the prospect of hospital. She had already been to the priory many times as a teenager. She hated it there. She hated herself for hating it. Why was hospital this constant contradiction? Why were people constantly mentioning it as a possibility?

Julie spoke softly, quietly, only very vaguely peering out of her protected shell. She did not know how to speak to this man, this gentle giant. She did not know how to express herself, say what was really on her mind. She wanted to say how very afraid she was about the idea of going into hospital. Despite her social worker, her counsellor and her friends despairing with the doctor that it was necessary, Julie still did not want to get admitted. She was petrified.

"You are very young for your age. Very young." His comments stung. Obviously he was saying she was stupid and immature. She was not normally like this. Normally she was more confident and outgoing, not this vulnerable mess she was in this office. In this office she was merely a child, but in the outside world she had been a teacher and been in charge of thirty children. But in here she was jelly. This was not her. The woman he was seeing and treating was not her. It was someone else. She felt disassociated from her body. But as he spoke and treated her like a child, then she had no choice but to abide. It was him just as much as her. He remarked how he saw her like one of his daughters who was a bit lost in the big wide world, and she laid down to his words.

"Julie, Julie, you silly child, what are you doing?" Mrs Kenny screamed at her, "get out from under the table and do your adding!" Julie did not move. She could not concentrate on the jumble of numbers on the page, and she did not want to. Nobody was going to make her. Mummy, mummy, I don't like school. Mummy cries again. Pulls me in her lap and tells me her secrets. Don't talk to anyone. Don't trust anyone. Nobody is your friend and everyone is mean. Only I am your friend. Only my mummy is my friend.

Chapter 2

Borderline; the diagnosis that psychiatric staff hate the most.

Entering the big doors of the hospital is the unknown. Julie's fears of what will happen to her are numbed and fragmented. She is walking in a dream, surrounded by nothing and surrounded by chaos. The world is something to fear and yet to conquer. She is in hospital, she must be ill. Very ill. Or else just a time waster.

"Hello, my name is Edith," said a beautiful Russian girl. She is tall and slim and is too pretty. Never trust anyone too pretty. They just have a better disguise than most. "Here, let me show you your room." Julie follows her down a long wooden hall. It is not unpleasant, nor is it nice. It just was. There were a few strange smells consummating of hospital food and disinfectant, plus a unique musty smell she had never experienced.

The room was simple and unwelcoming. There was a bed covered in plastic, and a tiny wardrobe that looked dirty and sticky. A few sweet wrappers were stuck to the shelves and on the floors. Julie wrinkled her nose in disgust, unwilling to put her clothes away in such filth. There was a bedside table there, and when Julie opened the door she saw two pill bottles and a small piece of glass. She picked up the glass and put it in her pocket, and called Edith back to show her the pills. She genuinely appeared to be shocked, then tried to explain it, as if it was her fault and she had literally put them there herself. Still numb, Julie shrugged her shoulders and sat on her bed. Edith had to look through her belongings, picking out creams, her razor and phone charger. Her independence was robbed.

On a Knife's Edge

When this was done, Edith left. Julie had nothing left to do but try and find her bearings. Where was she? How long would she be here for? What was going to happen now? She ventured down the hallway to find out.

A middle aged woman and a younger looking man were sitting at a table. The boy was hunched over, head in his hands and a twinkle in his eye. The woman was large and loud. "Hello, my name's Marian. Are you depressed?"

Julie shrugged. "No, I'm ok." The man and woman laughed.

"Sit down and start making friends," Marian ordered. Julie obeyed. She asked the man what his name was, but she could not understand. It sounded foreign, a bit like Borat. She told him so, never for a moment thinking that one day they would be good friends. He smiled and shook his head. Julie instantly relaxed and smiled back. She joined in the bantering conversation, and almost forgot she was supposed to be ill and depressed, until Edith reappeared.

"Julie, the doctor will see you now." Julie's insides froze in fear, and she silently pleaded with the world that the doctor would be kind, approachable and nonjudgmental. She went in and came out again, but if you asked her she would not be able to tell you anything that happened. Edith was shaking her head at her, disapproving. It wrenched Julie's heart. Why are you looking at me like that? What have I done? Julie was distraught. Edith pulled her aside into a little kitchen. "Now, I am not one for game playing. If you feel like hurting yourself you come and tell me. I don't play games," she repeated. She spoke at such high speed she must have been able to get through one hundred words a minute. She spoke perfect English with her

Russian accent. Shall I tell her my grandparents are Russian? No, she doesn't deserve to know.

Julie sat on her bed and looked at her arm. Blood was soaking up through the bandage. The small piece of glass was left on the side. The nurse was standing above her, waving her disapproving finger in her face.

"Do you think that looks pretty? Do you think your arm looks nice? Look at all those scars! What a waste of a life. A beautiful, young, intelligent girl like you, destroying herself like this." Julie said nothing. She sat looking down into her hands, so ashamed she could only wish to disappear. Tears welled up in her eyes, but she refused to let the nurse see. She would not give the nurse such satisfaction. "Well, Julie, aren't you going to say anything?" Julie had nothing to say to her. How could she begin to explain it to someone who was not interested in understanding?

It is hiding the scars that prove most difficult. I wear long sleeves even when it is so hot outside and my arms stick to my clothes like Clingfilm. Or perhaps I can walk around with a cardigan draped over my arm looking like a security blanket. And yet still I may be caught, just sometimes when I least expect it. I roll my sleeves up to do the washing up, I move my arm to reach something, a sleeve will roll up the hidden arm and I see the look on the face of whoever I am talking to. That look of shock, of fear, of pity. But how can they understand?

The trauma of an argument with him the almighty can send me to do this. It is a relief, I feel like my chest is going to explode and then I do it and a calm and flowing river surrounds my body giving me warmth and comfort. The shaky and unclear thoughts that mingle around in a

On a Knife's Edge

knotted twine in my head start floating. The night of the living dead surrounds me and holds me tight until it can be released. My breathing gets faster, my eyes get wider. Rapidly taking in air that refuses to come until I release it. The pain, the weight, the sorrow all needs to be let loose.

I used to think I was crazy. A shattered piece of glass can be my hero. A shiny object reflecting in the sun used to chop my carrots and grate my cheese can be used for such harmony. Some people may look upon my stripy arm and think of violence but it is the opposite. It is a form of neutrality.

When I try to see reason and stop it all the voices inside the walls scream at me. It is yelling so much and the words are spinning around my head. He is the one in charge and he can bully me because I am smaller than him. He tortures me and haunts me from whatever point in the house I try and hide. However hard I put my hands over my ears he can still get inside my ear drums and give me commands. He tells me how much better he will make me feel if I do it, just one more time.

Eventually I give in to these threats. Everyone is in bed so it is alright and safe or I can always go and run to the toilets where the door is locked, for the action requires privacy. I will never be caught. I open the door and sit beside it on the crouched wooden floor and bring the small piece of glass to hand. It may be cold but it can make such a hot singe on my arm. In one quick movement it is done, but often it is not enough. There is not enough warmth and not enough relaxation, so I repeat the action several times until I sit back and feel satisfied. I must go and fetch a tissue and mop it up before it drips, but before I do I take a look at those gorgeous red streaks that will be tattooed on my arm forever.

Myles was also an inpatient and Julie liked Myles, and Myles liked Julie. Liked being the operative word. They'd had a fight, and Myles was angry with her. Julie had cut herself again and Myles could not handle it. He was absolutely fuming with her, sending her angry text messages. Julie could not cope. She looked at the last message and was over swept by such intimidating confusion that she closed the lid in sadness. She did not know why he was so angry with her, why he was talking to her like that. The whole world was one big secondary school made up of bullies and angry teenagers, and the psychiatric nurses were there to rule the naughty school girls. St Trinion girls are the world of psychiatric wards. That was how they made Julie feel.

"Why are you so angry with me? Why are you telling me off?" Julie pleaded with him.
"You didn't come and talk to me. You didn't even give me a chance to help you. You cut yourself twice in such a short space of time. You'll never get out of here if you keep this up. How can I help you if you won't help yourself? I can't be outside your door twenty four hours." He said this in somewhat disgust, and with a bittersweet distaste. Julie's head was swimming. Why was he talking to her like this? What had she done that was so wrong? She didn't understand. She hated the way he was talking to her.
"You're just telling me off!" she cried to him, "Why are you talking to me like that? Stop telling me off."
Myles's face went a stronger shade of red. He clenched his fists in fury and said, "I can't talk to you when you're like this," and stormed off.

Julie felt unusually calm, mainly due to her lack of understanding. He texted her a moment later: I don't know what to do. I have got my own shit to deal with today. I don't need yours as well. Julie did not know how to respond, only saying that she understood but he did not need to take it out on her. But it didn't end there. He texted back: I haven't taken anything out on you. I walked out in self preservation! Big difference - balls in your court. I'm sorry I'm human not a saint. This last text was even more muddling. Julie stared at the phone, and went and picked up the glass. Almost in anger, almost as if she needed to prove to herself she was in control. If she wanted to, she would self harm. She needed that power, that choice. And nobody was going to take it away. The doctor would help her to stop, but he understood. He understood her need and her addiction. And if she had to prove to the world that she could cut if she wanted to, then she would cut. Over and over again. Watch the blood. Whip the glass across her flesh until it stung. It would sting and as it bled she would feel the tension bleeding away from her body. Self preservation - a wonderful thing.

The next morning, Julie decided not to get up for breakfast. She was hurt by the comments of the nurse last night, and Myles's words stung in her memory. As she lay in bed she heard the noisy chatter of the kitchen situated just outside her door. Pass me the milk please love. Any spoons? Where's the fucking sugar? Were just some of the things she heard. She tried to block out these sounds, put her fingers in her ears. Put the pillow over her head. Made an effort to stuff rolled up bits of Kleenex between her ears, but this did nothing. She sat up in bed, sleepy eyed, and felt she was fighting a losing battle. She was not going to get any more sleep, that was certain. Perhaps she would have more luck getting out of bed and having a bath.

She scooped up her bag of soaps, shampoos and

moisturisers and her intended outfit for the day and trotted out. The bathroom door was locked. She caught sight of Georgina and grabbed her arm.

"Can you unlock the bathroom door, please?" She asked Georgina.

Georgina shook her head apologetically. "No, sorry. The plumbing has gone a bit crazy today. There's no cold water. You can't use the bath, or the shower for that matter."

"But how are we supposed to wash? When can we use it again?"

Georgina shrugged her shoulders. "I don't know. Perhaps it will be sorted in a few days. In the mean time, if you grab a couple of paper towels you can wash yourself in the sink." She began walking off, muttering to another nurse about the amount of depressed people who did not want to wash anyhow. Too depressed to think of hygiene! But this was not the case for Julie. Julie felt dirty and smelly if she did not wash, and the idea of waiting at least a couple of days for a shower sent frills of panic down her spine. In these moments, which were becoming more and more frequent, Julie longed to just disappear. She ran back to her room, anger pending up from within. She longed to scream and cry. She sat down and tried to sob, but was met only with dry tears of emptiness. She could not cry! She could not even force herself to cry, despite feeling so cut up inside. Instead, she went to her secret piece of glass and cut deep into her arm, but it was not enough. The cut was too superficial; there was no blood, no inside damage. She repeated the action but still felt no satisfaction, so she curled up on the bed and willed sleep to come. At last she was able to escape.

She had felt so strange on her first day in Watford. You'll be in hospital one, two, three nights at the most, but no more, Keith from the CAT team had said. But that was nearly five weeks ago now. Julie remembered the strange sensation, the unease of the unknown. What would life be like in here? What did they do all day? Well, since the nurses were unwilling to share this information, she decided the only way to find out was to ask the patients.

A middle aged man was continuously walking round the corridors with a cup of tea. He looked normal, sane. Not on another planet like some of the other patients muttering to themselves. Julie's new focus was on him. She tried to make conversation. "What's your name?" she said in such a timid voice, it reminded her of a child curiously approaching a stranger.

"Rob. What's yours?" he had kind eyes, but with a touch of sadness. His big fluffy fleece made Julie want to wrap her arms around him, but she relented.

Julie asked, "What do you do in the day here?"

"Well, you get up for breakfast, take meds, and then the rest of the day is totally up to you."

"You mean, there are no groups or therapy or anything like that?"

Rob looked thoughtful. "Well, occasionally some people might do some art, but not really. You just do what you want to do."

"But what are the options?" Julie was starting to feel helpless.

"There aren't any options really. Just sitting or walking around. Are you allowed out?"

"I don't know. I'll ask." Julie went over to the nurse's office and knocked on the door.

"Be with you in a moment," was the response. The nurse sitting there did not even turn around, but kept his back to her.

"I just wanted to know if I'm allowed out at all," Julie felt her voice trailing off and leaving her behind.

The nurse turned around abruptly. "I said, I'll be with

you in a minute!"

"Oh, sorry," Julie felt silly apologising. She went and sat down on a window ledge near the office. Half an hour later, and three games of Sudoku later, the nurse was still sat at the computer. Julie let out a long sigh, and got up, and started following Rob around.

The evening improved somewhat. All the patients were sitting around the tables, chatting and laughing. Julie sat with Borat, Rob and a few others. There was chatter and jokes, and people generally seemed to be in a good mood. The nurses were still shut away in the office, and it was only from talking amongst the other patients that Julie felt any healing was going on.

In the times before being admitted to hospital, Julie had made frequent visits to the emergency department. She was scared, so scared. The blood was soaking through everything. The tissues had disintegrated in the liquid, even the towel was not holding it in. She was pressing as hard as possible. She phoned Anna up, slightly hysterical.

"It's bleeding so much. I'm scared."

"Do you need me to take you to hospital?"

"Yes. But I'm so scared. What if they put me in hospital?"

"Well, don't worry about that now. Listen, I'm just going to have my dinner. I should be with you by eight at the latest."

Julie looked at the clock. It was a quarter to seven. She looked at all the blood soaked towels, and humbly agreed to wait for Anna. She sat and waited with a heavy black coat on so that the blood would not show. Her mother was on the phone and had not noticed. Not an unusual thing! Julie felt a mixture of gratitude to Anna, but at the same time she felt hurt that Anna had not come instantly. Immediately she felt guilty for thinking this. She allured herself to wait and to be a good little girl who was grateful for any act of kindness.

Anna arrived and let out a gasp when she saw how much blood there was. So much blood! Anna could not believe it, and hurried Julie into the car.
"I don't mean to be insensitive, but can you try not to get blood on my car please," was the first thing that was said. Julie agreed. She could not condemn Anna for saying that. Julie was such a pain, and an inconvenience to the world, that was certain.

In the hospital Anna immediately asked the receptionist for a bandage. The response was not positive. "She'll need to wait to be seen by triage."
"But she's bleeding everywhere. She's bleeding all over the floor and all over the seats!" The receptionist merely shrugged her shoulder, and handed her a paper towel. Julie laughed at this mockery, and just let the blood flow.
Anna marched over to reception. "Excuse me, excuse me, but this is ridiculous. She is bleeding everywhere!" The receptionist made a comment about waiting turns, and in the end Anna gave up. In her head she imagined spitting at the nurses, throw the blood stained towels in their faces. She refrained from using a few four letter words, as she realised this may only hinder their situation.

Julie started to feel dizzy. The ground marginally started to sway from side to side, and Julie's head felt a flush of heat. Next thing she knew she was being propped up by Anna. Anna's voice was faint and far away. "Can someone help......?" Julie felt herself being propped up on the chairs. A nurse was making her sit up. Julie opened her eyes.
"There we go, all better. Now stay here please," the

nurse walked off and left the pair of them sitting there, Anna supporting Julie's head which felt a bit like a bowling ball at that moment. Anna's voice was raging about the state of affairs, but Julie just closed her eyes and imagined she was another person. A happy person, running in the fields with long blonde hair blowing in the wind. She was thrown back to reality when the doctor started to inject her with anaesthetic before giving her some quintessential blue stitches.

"Right, now Julie," the doctor put his hands on his knees, swivelled round on his chair and stared at her, "I'd like to refer you over to the CAT team."

"What's that?"

"Crisis and Assessment team. They will just talk to you and find out ways they can help. Hospital or home help."

Panic raged within Julie's stomach when she heard these words. Hospital? She did not want to be going to hospital; that she was sure of. She shook her head and tried to excuse herself, but the doctor was persistent. Reluctantly, Julie agreed. Anna stayed with her.

Julie began to joke around with Anna. She had gone beyond the point of despair, and the only direction now was up. They both made themselves as comfortable as was possible in the corridor. After another three hours, they were promoted to an actual room with comfier chairs. Julie's eyes were heavy; it was getting on to three in the morning. Then Anna got the call from Elizabeth.

Elizabeth used to call herself Julie's best friend. At one point, Julie had seen her almost every day. They had shopped, cooked, slept and even gone on holiday with each other. They loved each other's company and Julie loved the sound of Elizabeth's machine gun laugh. But then Julie got ill, she was depressed. Elizabeth got married to a highly unpleasant man who found it totally acceptable to shout and verbally abuse Julie. As a result, their friendship had fluctuated to almost non-existence. But Elizabeth still felt she had the right to interfere and hurt Julie as much as possible.

"No, no, I don't mind staying," she heard Anna saying into the phone, "I can't just leave her! Look, I have to go, Julie's getting upset with this conversation. No, I think I can make up my own mind about whether I can stay here or not. Yes, fine, good night." Julie felt her anxiety levels rising and held onto Anna's sleeve in terror.
"Why, why did she want you to leave me here? Why didn't she care?" Julie could not believe it. All those hours of friendship had truly disappeared, and she saw how cruel the world really was.

Eventually, the CAT team arrived. By this point, Julie was so exhausted, she could barely speak. It turned out the only thing the CAT team did was to give Julie a phone number she could call out of hours. When Julie went to type the number in her phone, she found the number was already there.

Chapter 3

It was going to be a fun day out! A day out with her mum. Julie had been in hospital nearly six weeks now, and her mother had never once come to visit. But she was coming today to take her out. They were going to go to the cinema to see Slumdog Millionaire - it was supposed to be brilliant, won some academy awards. Julie was looking forward to the time to spend together.

The day started off well. Her mother came to get her, and Julie had just finished her painting. She was enjoying the time she spent in the art rooms and was really discovering a hidden talent. When her mother laid eyes on her paintings she gasped in admiration at the paintings.
"Wow, you really are so talented," she beamed with pride. Julie showed her the rest of the paintings that were hung up on her wall. Each was met with approving sounds.

The cinema trip was successful, and Julie and her mother were enjoying the laughter of their relationship. Once home, Julie decided to quickly cook them both some pasta before her mother took her back to the hospital. Unfortunately an unexpected visitor arrived half way through their meal, Julie's sister Jenna.

Jenna came in. She was in floods of tears. She put her head in her hands and announced very dramatically that she "could not go on." She had been feeling very bad and had asked her mother to go with her to see the doctor, but her mother had refused on account of the day that was planned with Julie. Julie felt bad for her sister and tried to make her feel better.
"Are you still seeing your psychologist?" Julie inquired.

On a Knife's Edge

"Yes," Jenna's tone sounded harsh, but Julie did not catch on.

"Well, I'm sure if you start telling her how you feel..."

Jenna stood up, knocking the chair flying behind her. She pointed an accusing finger at Julie. "I cannot believe they let a stupid, attention seeking person like you into hospital, and they tell me there is nothing wrong with me. You are a nasty, game playing little bitch."

Julie stopped eating. "Take me back to hospital RIGHT NOW!" she demanded. She ran upstairs to fetch her bag and shoes, but Jenna was not finished with her.

"I know about you. I know all about you. You pretend to get depressed, you pretend to hear voices in the walls, but it's all lies. You want to be in hospital so that you have all the attention..."

Julie interrupted her. "Well, Jenna, if you can't cope anymore why don't you just kill yourself. Go and fucking kill yourself!"

The next moments all happened in a speedy, disjointed eruption. Jenna started attacking Julie, pulling her hair and scratching her. Unfortunately for Jenna, Julie was a lot stronger and was able to fight back quite easily. Their mother was hysterically trying to stand in-between, but with not much luck.

Julie could not take anymore. "Take me back now!" But her mother refused. Julie grabbed her car keys and started announcing she was going to drive herself back. But her mother stood at the door.

"You can't go back. Not like this. I can't let you leave like this." Julie pushed her mother out the way, but she would not move. Jenna was screeching in her ear, threatening her, tormenting her. Julie ran into the corner to phone Myles.

"What do you expect me to do about it?" Myles responded. Julie hung up on him; he was clearly not going to help. She had no choice; she had to call the police.

"My sister is attacking me and my mum won't let me out of the house," Julie spluttered into the phone. Jenna snatched the phone out of her hand and continued her torments.

Eventually Julie ran out to the car, half throwing her mother out of the way. Jenna ran after her, willing her to continue hitting her. Her mother stood behind the car, refusing to let her go. Furious, Julie got out the car and screeched at her mother to get out of the way. Jenna pursued with shouting insults at Julie until Julie turned round and punched her in the eye. A police car pulled up and stopped. Julie and her mother ran into the house, leaving Jenna and the police.

Back in the house, Julie's mother started to play martyr. "I don't deserve to be treated like this. I should never have had children. I should have had an abortion."

Julie could not believe her ears. All her mother could think about was herself. After everything she had just been through, listening to the poisoning words of her sister, feeling the venom of her fists, and her mother could only think of herself. This was too much. Julie wanted out. She wanted to make damn sure nobody could hurt her anymore.

She grabbed a large pack of paracetamol, and took it upstairs. She started to swallow them, one after the other. After she had reached seventeen, she heard a knock at the door.

"Julie, it's the police, open the door." Unwillingly, she opened it. They picked up the packets of pills. "How many have you taken?" Without saying a word, Julie handed her the empty packets. The policewoman spoke into her walkie talkie. "Ambulance please, overdose."

Downstairs, Julie sat with a policeman, whilst her

mother explained what had happened. Fortunately for Julie, her mother told the story in her favour. She heard her mother saying, "Julie was actually being quite nice to Jenna. But Jenna was awful to her."

"Your sister has a black eye, but it seems like it was all in self-defence," the policewoman explained, "don't worry, you won't get in trouble for it."

The ambulance crew arrived and took some blood, blood pressure and pulse. All was fine. Julie was physically fine. "Will you take me back to hospital please?"

The policewoman asked Julie if she would mind her mother taking her back to hospital as they were very busy, but the paramedic took the policeman aside. "I'm sorry; I don't think that would be a good idea." In the end the policewoman agreed to take Julie back to hospital. Jenna was sitting in another police car, and as Julie backed out of the drive with her police pair, she saw the evil, black stare of her sister following her as she reversed out of the driveway.

Julie woke up the next morning and felt wretched. Her head was throbbing, her stomach was moaning at her, but most of all her heart was aching. She felt isolated and depressed. She went to ask her nurse for an extra pill and went to sleep. She woke up at three in the afternoon, but her depression was still very much present. She lay on her bed, half asleep and in a dreamlike state, until she could not bear it anymore.

To try and rid the isolation, she phoned up her friend John. John had been amazing to her, visiting her every weekend without fail. He was such a busy person managing a whole computer company, doing volunteer work a few nights a week and studying part time for a Masters degree; yet he still found time to visit Julie. He would not abandon her.

John was an awkward chap; too tall, too dark, too cross eyed. His voice and posture reeked of the shyness he tried to prevail. He was slightly cocky and arrogant, but his heart was made of pure gold. When Julie needed a friend more than she needed anything else in the world, John was there at her doorstep.

When John walked into her hospital room, Julie flung her arms around him. She held him tight and did not want to let him go. He towered above her, awkwardly putting his arms back round Julie, before patting her on the head and pushing her away. You could almost hear the sounds of relief as she sat down and he sat comfortably half a metre away.

John listened as Julie recounted the events of the previous night. He sat with a leg crossed, stroking the stubble on his chin. "Hmm," was how he started, "not erm, not very nice at all. No, in fact it sounds all rather horrible." To an outsider he was mocking, but Julie knew his tones and his gestures. He was generally upset for Julie and felt his responsibility to cheer her up. He whipped out a small USB modem. "Look, pass me your laptop and I'll sort it so that you can connect to the internet." He was very proud of himself.

The internet...now Julie would have no excuse to be disconnected from the outside world. Was that good or bad?

Myles was being discharged from the hospital; he was going to Unicorn House. Unicorn House was a half-way house where he would be allowed to come and go as he pleased. There would be staff there in the day, but at night he would be on his own. It was a big step forward.

"I'll come and see you every day," he promised. He sounded sincere, but deep down they both knew that they would not be seeing each other every day. Julie would bet her life on it.

The bell rung to signal break time. Julie went out and scanned the playground for her little group of friends. We'll be friends forever... they had agreed at the weekend. They had all shook on it, and Julie felt so secure in this past. She spotted Lisa and Felicity over by the wall near to the entrance to the girls' toilets. She waved and started to walk over. As she approached them, Lisa and Felicity looked at each other. They picked up their bags and together they ran off, ran away from Julie. Julie was left there, watching. Watching her friends run away from her. It was from then that Julie began to hate herself.

Never trust anyone. You cannot trust anyone except me, your mother. I am the only one who will love you. DON'T TRUST ANYONE.

Julie had dry tears. She hated dry tears, the sort that were brewing but would not spill. It made her want to die. Oh, the blissful feeling of dying, to go to a place where nobody could hurt her. But how did she know? How did she know that if she died it would be better or worse? Or what if she tried to kill herself and it didn't work and she ended up paralysed or dying a long, slow, painful death? There were so many things to consider. But at the end of the day, she could not stand the pain. The pain of depression, of the torments she went through on the inside. The voices were shouting at her, telling her she was worthless and it was wrong that she was alive. She should not be alive, she should be dead. The agony of living was too strenuous. Each movement, each breath hurt her. She was immobilised, and death seemed like such a sweet relief. A delightful relief to the pain and voices confusing her in her head. She opened up the bottle of pills, and swallowed each pill one by one.

Chapter 4

It was the dire boredom that got to Julie sometimes on the ward. It was going on three months and Julie was starting to lose count. When there was nothing to do, nothing to fill up your time with. The people walked around like zombies, either depressed or crazy. But which was Julie? Where did she belong?

Beverly was crazy. She was in her late sixties, but thought she was in her late twenties. Her choice of fashion never stopped surprising her inmates. The bright pinks always seemed to clash with the vibrant silvers and golds. Her handbag looked like it had been ripped to shreds by a pack of wild dogs. Her hair was a desperate mess of hairclips and tangles. She never seemed to get it right. She had crazy swarming her like flies.

Her high-pitched throaty voice hit Julie in streams of shivers down her back. "Morning Julie, you look nice today. My mum was supposed to come today but she didn't but that's ok because Martin had a heart attack but he shouldn't have done that as there is nobody to feed the cat and my neighbour rung and told me this and I've been in tears all morning…"

Julie ran up the stairs muttering, "hi, Beverly," and disappeared up the stairs. Everybody felt sorry for her, thought it was a shame. But nobody had any time for her, not one person could get to her level of communication. Beverly continues to wander the corridors of the psychiatric ward, lonely and a symbol of avoidance for both staff and Patients.

What could she do to occupy her time? There was little choice. Her depression was elevated by her boredom, and her depression prevented her from engaging in any activity, thus making her more bored. A vicious cycle of emptiness.

As usual, Kerry came to her rescue by creating such a noise of disturbance, Julie felt knots inside her tightening with every yell, with every cry of anger Kerry used. Kerry was angry, and when Kerry was angry the entire unit would know. Doors would be slammed, chairs thrown, black staff threatened. She terrified Julie, but at the same time her expressions of irritation marvelled her. When Julie was angry, she kept it all within, took it out on herself. Kerry was able to express this anger, though not in a nice way because it upset others. Julie contemplated a healthy way of letting out pain, but was met with a blank thought.

She sat beside one of the student nurses. "What do you do when you're angry?" she asked Rocky, the Philippine student nurse.

"I go to my room for some me time."

"What do you mean by me time?"

"Oh, you know, I go to my room, look at porn and jerk off."

Julie nodded. She would not be asking him again.

Johnn had been her only friend, the only one she could rely on. He'd come to see her weekly, and speak to her daily. You can call me anytime; I'll always be here for you. Julie believed him and put her faith into him. It would be at least a whole year before he let her down too.

It was Friday. It was exactly one week since her huge emasculating row with her sister, and Julie was terrified it was going to happen again. She knew her sister came to the hospital on Fridays for art therapy, today. Julie was convinced her sister was out to get her, to kill her. She went to inform Rocky of her fears.

On a Knife's Edge

"She is going to kill me. I know she is. She tried to kill me last Friday and I had to call the police. She is going to try to kill me!" Julie pleaded with him. Rocky looked at her like a foreign object, nodded his head in agreement. Patronising idiot!

John - she would tell John. He was sure to listen. She called him up in a frantic state.

"She's going to kill me. I know my sister is going to come and kill me today," she almost shrieked into the phone.

"Look, Julie, you got to stop this. She's not going to kill you. She might be angry with you and hit you, but that hardly means she is going to kill you."

He was not listening to her. She had to make him believe it.

"No, you don't understand, she really is going to try and kill me. You have to come and pick me up. Please come and pick me up?"

"No, I can't do that I'm afraid, I'm at work. They'll never let you out if you start saying things like that. You got to start dealing with things by yourself. You can't rely on me all the time. I got my own life to lead."

Julie felt his words punching her in the stomach and sending her heart rolling into space. "You mean you don't want to be my friend anymore," she said in a tiny voice.

"No, I didn't say that. You just got to start dealing with things yourself and not rely on me. You understand don't you?"

Julie could not utter anything comprehensible. She felt too hurt. She murmured good bye and then hung up. Then she took out her stash of glass and repeatedly cut herself over and over, watching the blood trickling down her arm.

She could hear them. They were talking, louder and more evil each minute. They were trying to kill her. They were hidden in the walls, voices distant and undistinguished. You should die. It is WRONG that you are alive. You should not be here, you should be dead. Dead. Dead. Julie covered her ears and screamed. She ran out her bedroom onto the landing, where Neera was sitting, staring at her. The sounds were ringing in her ears, crawling into her veins. She could not remove them, however far she ran or however hard she pressed her delicate hands against her eardrums.

She started to bang her head against the wall, over and over so that the sounds would go away. Eventually they went, and she sat there, dizzy and confused. Neera was still watching her, lips uneven, eyes shifting. "Julie, why the hell are you banging your head at the wall?" she asked in a heavy Indian accent. Julie said nothing. She gazed back at Neera, still woozy and unable to say anything of meaning.

She wanted someone to help her, comfort her, and show her a small act of kindness. She was desperately pleading with Neera, but it soon became clear she was going to get nothing in return for her distress but a snarl.

Julie felt tears of rage burning her eyelids. Once again, Myles had let her down. Every day this week, she had been made promises of visits and outings, and each day they were cancelled. This was the last straw; she had been looking forward to going out that day, really excited. But he had cancelled on her again, saying he was not good company today. This time, she refused to text back. Refused to let him control her, make her sad. He was breaking her heart into tiny shreds and she had to protect herself. She had to let him go.

But it was difficult. She missed him. The way he hugged her, sent her sweet text messages. But that was in the first few weeks when Julie was a novelty. All he wanted was sex, he did not need anything else. His promises of friendship were a harsh reality of rejection. Julie started to lose faith in the world and the people in it. She cut herself for the fourth time that day.

She ran out the room, slightly panicking. It was deep this time, she was sure. The bandage wasn't holding it, the tissues were soaking through. She opened the door and yelled for James. Another nurse, Rhea was sitting on a chair outside the living room.

"Did you cut yourself? Julie, I'm talking to you, did you cut yourself?" Julie did not want to talk to this woman bellowing at her. She grew frightened and started to run, panic and sweat surrounding her. The nurse followed her and Julie picked up speed.

"Where's James? Where's James?" she kept yelling, ignoring Rhea's orders to stop. James came running out the staff room, and stopped Julie in her tracks.

"No, Julie, that's not on. You can't run around dripping blood all over the carpet, it's against health and safety. You'll have to go with Rhea to clean that up."

As Rhea led Julie to the medicine bay James whispered loud enough for Julie to hear, "you were right," and she silently took out the necessary bandages and did not glance at Julie once.

Chapter 5

Myles had hurt Julie for the last time that day. She had had enough of his cruelty towards her. She recalled in her mind over and over again how he treated her.

He's just texted me to cancel on me again. I was so looking forward to going out for lunch with him; I was counting on that activity for the day. She should have known he would cancel; he always cancelled. He was so selfish. She asked for an extra pill of quetiapine and went to sleep all morning. The room reeked of hurt and disappointment.
She was not going to text. She wouldn't do it. Why should she? He didn't care how much he'd hurt her. He didn't care how upset and let down she felt. She was not going to let him in again.
But of course he texted her the next day: "are you still my friend? Sorry been so depressed lately. I know you don't give a damn." How could he say that? Am I evil? I am an evil person who does not deserve to live because everybody, absolutely everybody, hates me. Why is my life like this? I need to text back: "I'm sorry I was evil."

They made up, gave the impression of being friends again. Arranged to meet up the next day; Myles wanted Julie to accompany him to make a business deal. He needed Julie there, needed a favour. Julie felt like an obedient sheep and followed him.
He started on her. "Why are you still in hospital? Do you stay there for the attention? It's pathetic!" Julie did not comment. She fought back choking tears. He didn't stop there. "I think you should just tell your mum what a fucking awful mother she is! Why don't you just tell her instead of being so nice to her? It's a fucking Joke!" Julie started to stick up for herself, explain that her

mother needed her help. She needed Julie to be the strong one. Myles said everything with his loud silence.

"Your driving is bloody awful. I can't believe you coast it's so dangerous. You're going to cause an accident one of these days…." Julie could not hold it in. She started some quiet sobbing, not knowing how to cope with feeling so low.

The next day Julie thought about how he had treated her and she did not like it. She wanted to tell him, to stop him. She texted him very clearly: "it really hurts me when you make mean comments about me. I don't think it's very nice." She sat on her bed, staring at her phone. She was anticipating a response, calculating the minutes in her head. Her phone beeped back: "Well, find yourself someone else. I don't want to be your friend anymore." Julie had anticipated an angry, defensive response, but she knew she could not play his games anymore. She never won these games; she always lost. But not this time: "I'm sorry you feel like that. I was just being honest. I hope you find a better friend. Good bye."

At first she felt relief. Relief that she would not have to endure the nasty comments. No longer could he hurt her. But then she just felt sad. Not sad for Myles, just sad that she realised she could not understand the people in this world. Why are people such shits?

The next day was too much for Julie to bear. What was the point in being alive when the world was such a cruel place to be in? She was ashamed to be a part of the human race; she was ashamed to be alive in this world. She lay in bed and wished she was dead. A moment later, someone switched on the light in her bedroom and said, "breakfast!" Julie felt pissed off, but also silently thankful. She now had a purpose, to get up and eat breakfast.

She put on her dressing gown, and slowly plodded along the dirty wooden stairs that had a mixed smell of food and urine. One of the Patients urinates on the ground. She had also been known to shit on the floor. Funny thing is, she used to be a nurse, and a good nurse at that. Alcohol could change a person dramatically.

Julie picked up the flimsy plastic bowl, and put in her cereal. She had a plastic spoon and a plastic cup of tea to go with it. Funny thing was, when everything was made of plastic, everything tasted of plastic.

After breakfast Julie began her routine. She went back to her room, cleaned her teeth and flossed until her gums bled, because she liked to cause herself physical pain of any kind. Then she sat on her bed. Last time she saw the doctor, she was told that the next time she had an urge to cut, she should wait fifteen minutes. Then she would write it down in her log. Her mood before, her mood after, and the triggers. She kept this log religiously; though she was pretty convinced nobody would have time to look at it.

Then she started to wonder round on the ward. It was Wednesday, and there was pottery in the morning. Great! She remembered that Myles would be there, and she felt her stomach tightening up. What would he be like? Would he be nasty? Should she tell anyone? She went up to a nurse and asked if she could talk to her. "Give me a minute and I'll get back to you," she said. The nurse did not get back to her.

Mary-Anne, a student nurse, was standing in the living room grooming her nails. Julie gently tugged her. "Myles has upset me..." she told Mary-Anne all about the nasty texts and the feelings of hurt and upset she had been through afterwards. Mary-Anne actually listened.

"It's tough, you know," she sympathised, "some

people are just like that. Sometimes you just got to rely on yourself. Don't worry; I'll come to pottery with you. Just come find me."

At medication time, Julie stood and waited. Each patient had to have their medication and form an orderly queue. The waiting time was painfully slow. The nurses seemed to take at least ten minutes putting the medication into the cups, slowly counting each milligram and recording it on the notes. Julie often wondered if they were manufacturing the pills behind the counter.

When Julie finally got to the front, the nurses decided it was time to have a little look at what medication they needed to order. She stood and was ignored. She pinched herself to check she was real, then politely inquired as to whether she should come back.

"No, just sit down there and wait," the nurse responded. Once again feeling rejected and uncared for, Julie just walked away. Some things were more trouble than they were worth.

At ten thirty, it was time for pottery. Julie peered in through the window, her heart skipping a beat when she saw Myles sitting there. She had half expected him not to show up, but there he was, and Mary-Anne was nowhere to be seen. She stood at the door, too hesitant to go in.

When Mary-Anne walked past, she grabbed her hand and walked into the clay room. She sat down with Julie, who was shaking and woozy from the panic. And then she started to relax and enjoyed making some figures with Mary-Anne beside her. Mary-Anne tried to make a person, and Julie kept finding sexual innuendos to everything she was making. That looks like a pair of boobs! That looks like a sperm! And the two of them giggled like school girls. Myles glanced at her now and then and said nothing. Julie continued to laugh, but felt the ever negative presence of Myles near her and by the end, she felt close to tears. She went into her room to allow herself to cry, but as usual they refused to flow.

Chapter 6

She had the internet! John had given her something to use for the internet. A little black device known as a modem USB, and now she was able to communicate with the outside world. The void of Myles's departure from her life would start to fill up again. She went on chatting websites and chatted with her friends.

There was somebody she missed now he was gone. Cyrus. Cyrus walked in one day when Julie was eating her lunch. He was different to the others. He had a shaved head with huge tattooed spiders, and long baggy clothes. He immediately sparked Julie's interest and she nostalgically remembered her teenage years in Camden Town. When she was in the sixth form she had spent many hours with her friends by the river, smoking weed and drinking alcohol and popping pills. It was wrong, so wrong. She had loved every minute of it. She had been a part of something; she had a part to play in a crowd. She was the youngest, the cutest, the most innocent who needed people to teach her about the art of making a spliff. She wore clothes that were far too big for her size ten body. Big jumpers with System of a Down and Metallica. Huge jeans that flared from her legs. But she was so happy with her little group.
Cyrus look took her back to those relaxed and joyous times in Camden Town where she had fitted in, if only for the brief moment before they all realised she was an academic and she went off to study at a top London university, leaving behind life's loafers. Julie wanted to go back to them, but never quite found her way.

Cyrus stumbled around, half blinded by the light and buzzing of people. He looked heavily drugged, almost fighting to stay awake. Julie watched him drag himself across the dining room, but on his way she touched his arm slightly.

"Hi, I'm Julie," she said shyly. It was nice to talk to new people, just to take the edge out of that fear and loneliness.

He shook her hand. "I'm Cyrus."

Cyrus and Julie became inseparable. He was her rock. He was so kind, so thoughtful and tender to Julie's woes. He was cheerful and smiley. But what was wrong with him? On the surface he appeared to be fine, a normal guy hanging out with friends. On the inside he was broken, afraid to leave his flat and bereaved at his mother's death. The most dangerous aspect to him was that he was not afraid to die. He would quite happily torch himself just to prove a point. This terrified Julie.

When Cyrus discharged himself Julie was left in despair. She cried softly into her pillow that night, the tears were not afraid to freely flow. In her vivid dreams Cyrus covered himself in oil, took out a lighter and lit himself on fire. Julie screamed and tried to save him, but her hair caught fire. She woke up screaming. A nurse popped his head in and told her to be quiet, people were sleeping. She was too afraid to go to sleep; she got out of bed and wondered down the hall.

She sat down on a table near the nurses' office. She made herself a coffee and sat drinking it, trying to hide her feelings of sorrow and pain. Her chest was heavy and her eyelids flickered. She was to see the doctor today.

Trembling with fear and apprehension, she clock watched all day until her time had come to see the doctor. She slowly opened the door, following the nurse and sat down.

"Huh hmmm," the doctor cleared her throat, "I'm sorry but we're not ready. Please wait outside." Julie did not quite comprehend the doctor's words, and left the room sharply. Sickness started to lay itself at the pit of her stomach.

The doctor finally called her back. Julie was shaking so much she could not even utter a hello when she sat down in the room. Around her was the main doctor, two other doctors, a pharmacist, a psychologist, a mental health practitioner, a nurse and two members of the CAT team.

"We're sending you home this weekend, just to see how things go," the doctor said. Julie focussed her eyes on the doctor, nodding her head. She felt pleased, yet apprehensive.

She phoned around, and eventually her Cousin Pablo came to fetch her and take her home. Julie was chatty and tried to convince herself this was a positive thing. So why did she feel so sick to the stomach? Why did the hairs on the back of her neck quiver at the idea of seeing her family?

She got home and messed around. She watched television, she went on the internet, and she ate pop tarts. She distracted herself for a good few hours, until the depression started. It hit her like freezing cold water, and rapidly made its way round her body.

She could not stand the pain, the deep, deep pain rooted in her. It was unbearable, torture. She saw no point in being alive if she had to live with the pain. She actually began to believe that she would be better off dead.

She called Cyrus. Cried to him down the phone. He was suffering too. He was going to ask to be put back into hospital. He told her she needed to phone her CAT team and demand being placed back into hospital too. Julie called them, and they came round to her house. They looked at her, made comments. Julie rested her head on her hand and looked down at the ground. She did not speak, just the minimum words she could master. The CAT team left. They left her alone, and she went back to her room.

The pills were looking at her. The voices were chanting, take an overdose. Kill yourself. You would be better off dead. Death is the only way out, it is WRONG that you are alive. You should be dead. You should die. Julie picked up the bottle of pills and swallowed one after the other.

She was surprised to wake up Sunday afternoon, still alive, heart beating. She phoned the CAT team, sheepishly telling them what she had done. They came round, told her to pack a bag. She was going back to the hospital.

Her mother was sobbing away in the kitchen, crying out that people needed to feel sorry for her. They needed to help her, she could not live anymore, and she was a terrible mother. Julie ignored her and just kept thinking of Cyrus. I'm going to give you a big hug... he texted her.

But she had to stop off at A and E first, have some blood tests, make sure everything was alright. In cubicles a man tried to jump in her bed, stroking her breasts. Julie screamed. They took the man away, left Julie in a trance and terrified.

Eventually they brought her back to Cyrus, who caressed her and comforted her. There was something so loving at the way he cared, but how real was it? He did not want to become institutionalised, so he was leaving her again. In a few hours he was leaving her, but what Julie did not know was that he was leaving her for good.

"You'll never get rid of me, I'll be your best friend," was his promise before he left. He turned and left the hospital, not even looking back. Julie felt heartbroken.

She phoned him the next day. And the next. She was petrified he would kill himself, that she would lose him. He confided in her, told Julie he had a crush on her. Julie already knew, but she was not interested. Her head told her how wrong it would be, but her heart ached for him. She told him how unstable they both were, but in truth she loved him too much to watch him kill himself. She had to protect herself from that. But it did not matter, not when he promised to be her friend.

He did not keep in contact. He did not call her, did not text her. She was abandoned by a man she had loved so briefly. How could she be so wrong? How could she consistently be so wrong and trusting in such a heartless world? She occasionally tried to text him, but it was very clear he was not interested in her. She mourned his departure, clinging on to the memories.

Julie entered the mental health system at the age of fourteen. They said she had an eating disorder. Food ruled her life. Like many teenage girls, she did not want to be fat.

She sat bolt upright. She was sweating, her hands shaking. She found herself in the dark and immediately switched on the light. Her eyes shifted around, searching, looking. She knew they were there. She knew they were out to get her.

She was disgusted with herself for eating all that rubbish. For shoving her greedy mouth with biscuits, sweets, chocolate; basically anything she could get her hands on. She gobbled them down like she had a gun held there, forcing her. She was going to die tomorrow and this was her last bit of pleasure.

But it was all wrong. She felt so disgusted with herself. She did not deserve to eat so much, to have all these binges. It was wrong of her, vile. She looked at her repulsively large figure in the mirror. Looked at herself front ways, sideways. She tucked in her stomach, then puffed it out. She was so fat. She felt a wave of panic inside her. Her heart was beating. She could hear the blood from her ears thumping against her ear drums. You are so fat. You are so disgusting. You are so fat. You don't deserve to eat. Get rid of it. Get rid of it.

Julie dashed from her room, running away from the voices. She put her hands over her ears and tried to sing her calming song. Raindrops on roses and whiskers on kittens... she ran round and round, knowing she looked crazy and aware of awkward glances these are a few of my favourite things....die bitch die bitch fat fat fat fat....

She jolted into the toilets and locked the door, panting and leaning against the wall. She looked into the toilet and threw herself on the floor. She put her fingers down her throat and heaved. Nothing came up but phlegm. She tried again, desperately trying to get rid of the fattening food that was castrating her insides. She pushed her fingers further and further, making a mess of liquid bile on her fingers. A little food came up, but not enough. She stopped, sat back, slowly getting her breathe back. She hated herself for failing. She failed because she had eaten too much, and failed because she could not get rid of the food once she had eaten it. She was truly disgusted with herself.

She sat down on her bed and looked at the time. The doctor had given her the instructions. When she had the urge to cut herself, she was to wait twenty minutes. Then she would write down her mood before and after. It was to be recorded in her log. Julie's log. Julie's self-harm log!

She waited like a good girl. She sat and stared at her clock, waiting for the time to go on. But the time refused to go fast enough. It refused to go to the right time. It

On a Knife's Edge

seemed to take much long than five minutes to go to the next number. It was so slow; it took at least an hour for the twenty minutes to show on her phone. The phone was almost laughing at her. Teasing her that it was not keeping up with her urges. She picked it up and squeezed it, silently pleading with it to change.

Chapter 7

"Julie, do you know you have an appointment with the psychologist today at eleven?" Pergo the pedantic nurse informed her. Julie looked at her watch; ten forty five. She would never make it in time! If she had to walk to the clinic it would normally take her twenty minutes.

Without a moment to lose, she ran to her room, threw off her slippers and grabbed her handbag and dashed out of there. She power walked as she thought this might get her there faster than running. She looked at the time; five to eleven. She started to run, but shortly she had to stop. She was drawing in breath, her chest was heaving in the strain. She walked into the clinic at one minute past eleven.

"Please take a seat," the secretary asked her. Julie sat down, panting, feeling the rapid movements of her diaphragm going up and down, deeper and slower. She sat there for ten minutes before the psychologist asked her into his office.

She had seen him before in the assessment. He was a familiar face. He was in his mid forties, and had a huge forehead. He had kind wrinkles on his features, and eyes that looked straight at you. He asked about how she was feeling. The first memory that popped into Julie's head was the bust up with her sister. She recounted the events.

"I deal in CBT. We're going to try and explore things, but it needs to be a joint effort." Julie nodded, slightly intrigued. CBT? Cognitive behavioural therapy.

He drew a circle with a cross through the middle. "This is our hot cross bun, for obvious reasons. Now, we're going to separate this into four parts; behaviour, feelings, thoughts and biology. He put his pen down and looked Julie in the eye. "Now, let's take a scenario. A man comes home from work and his wife ignores him.

On a Knife's Edge

He gets depressed; he thinks his wife does not care about him and that the relationship is doomed. But if you look at it from another angle, his wife has had a bad day at work. Or she has had some bad news. His wife actually loves him very much, but was preoccupied with something else. If he had realised this, he would not have become depressed. Now, let's try and think about the episode with your sister. How did that make you feel?"

Julie, fascinated by this man, participated willingly in this task. She managed to put down angry, frustrated, scared, panicky and anxious. She looked at the list and remembered these feelings, but felt safe remembering them in the room. She began to work on the thoughts: I have to escape. I am worthless. I must be a terrible person. I can't cope. I want to die. Then she moved on to behaviour. She hit her sister; she tried to run away, she took an overdose. When it came to biology she found this more challenging, so the psychologist jumped in. She ended up noting that she was shaking, trembling and feeling sick. Stepping back Julie saw how all these linked, but the psychologist pointed out that her feelings led to her thoughts, which lead to her behaviour and biology. They were all entwined, and Julie needed to change one part to change the rest; her feelings.

Julie heard the familiar sound of her mobile ringing. She looked down and saw dad was calling her. She ignored him, clutched her palms around the speakers to stop the ringing. It stopped, but then started again. Unwillingly, she picked up the phone. She barely had time to say "hello" as her father barked at her down the phone.

"When are we going to see you? You never come home. We haven't heard from you in ages." Julie reluctantly agreed to make a trip home for lunch.

She started panicking the moment she hung up the phone and started getting ready. Her dad would be here to pick her up soon. The last thing she wanted was a confrontation so she dashed downstairs. But of course he was not there yet. She sat on the dirty wall, watching a woman from another ward smoking a cigarette. The smoke wafted out into the cold, freezing air. Fifteen minutes and two cigarettes later, her father pulled in.

She opened the door and sat down in the passenger seat, and despite the heating on she was met with an icier ambiance than outside. She did not know what to say, she felt her teeth gripping down together on her jaw like she had an invisible toffee wedged between her teeth. She waited for him to start.

"Your mother is desperately upset about what happened with you and your sister. Desperately upset!" He paused for emphasis, waiting for Julie to respond. She said nothing, but felt her jaw aching with the biting. She turned and looked out of the window, waiting for the next inevitable comment. "It was a complete disgrace what happened. You and your sister can never be in the same room again. It's such a shame. Such a shame, two sisters behaving like that. The neighbours had to call the police! They had to tell their children that the police were their friends and the screaming was rehearsing for a play! An absolute disgrace."

Silence. The silence of the car journey. It felt like this would never end. When she refused to respond he changed the subject. "So, when are they letting you out then?"

"I don't know yet. They don't want to let me out for some reason." Julie felt she had to portray that she wanted to come out, did not want to be there. She could not let him see any vulnerable side to her.

Her dad sneered. "Well, they must be keeping you in there for a reason. Are you still hurting yourself?" Julie's heart stopped beating, and she held her breathe at this comment. She mumbled an incomprehensible no, so her father continued his verbal diarrhoea. "Perhaps if you stop doing those silly things they'd let you out."

Smack bang round her neck. The air was tightening her neck. She was hurt. The evil forces were surrounding her, capturing her. They were banging, smacking, crashing around her body. Her body was wailing, tripping, crying. The tormented chants of the beasts. Kill yourself. Escape these sorts of people. All you have to do is find something of which to hang yourself, it would be so easy. Take an overdose, hang yourself with your belt. You don't have to be a part of this world anymore. You don't have to be a part of such misery. You can be free.

The car came to a roundabout and stopped. He changed up to fourth gear, stopped at some traffic lights. Julie watched with dull eyes.

I am evil. I am evil and I should die. It is wrong that I am alive I should not be alive I am a bad, terrible person who doesn't deserve to live I should be dead I need to kill myself I have to die stop torturing me why won't you leave me alone what have I done why am I so evil WHY DO I HAVE TO DIE?

Eventually they arrived home. She stammered out of the car, feeling like she was rolling through play equipment in a children's soft play. She rung on the door, face frozen, and jaws tightened, eyes dazed. The bell ring echoed in her ears, along with the loud clanging sound from her dad's key. The door opened in slow motion, and Julie walked in feeling like she was striding as a Charlie's angel. She was going to be confident in her own home.

She went to use a toilet that was not a hospital toilet. It was the toilet upstairs and was rarely used. There was no piss, no hairs, and no muck. Just a clean, cold, white toilet seat. She washed herself in a clean sink, without hand gel. She dried her hands on a soft towel; not on a paper towel. She looked at herself in the little cabinet mirror, and saw her teeth jammed together. She consciously loosened them, stood straight, then put her head in her hands and felt hot, stinging tears.

She went into her room and saw the piles of post lying around on her bed thrown there in a careless attempt. She opened them, one by one. Bills, notices, statements. Once they were read, they lay in a messy heap, envelopes and paper sticking out from under each other. Julie sat and stared at them, almost expecting them to move. She sat there for about fifteen minutes, shuddered then got up. She went downstairs and put on her sky plus television, and watched a sitcom she had recorded at Christmas time. Her parents were in the kitchen, speaking softly to each other. She was numb, silent. She was a ghost walking around in her own shadow, trapped from the rest of the world. Protected from pain and hurt in her invisible shell of nothingness.

She was called in for lunch, and unwillingly went into the dining room. She put on an air of cheerfulness, occasionally cracking a Joke. She allowed herself to laugh aloud, giving them the impression of a happy, well adjusted young lady, when inside she was fighting tears. She had to pretend to choke to cover up the tears, for at one point they threatened to spill. Her tears were a dripping tap, and eventually the drips have to spill over the edge.

The angry arguments with her mother were even more upsetting. It was about blame, about who was to blame for each other's pain. You did this, you said this. What was the point? Blame was not helpful, and it left Julie with such overwhelming feelings of loneliness, she was desperate to get back to the hospital to cut herself and relieve this tension.

She went into the dining room and put on the television. It felt strange, sitting on her own, in charge of the remote control. She flickered through the channels, not finding anything of interest. She wanted to go back to the hospital; she actually wanted to go back. She asked her father to drop her back.

"Why so early?" he sounded annoyed.

Julie had to make an excuse. She was not able to be honest and say she wanted to go back, she had to make out that she had to go back, like there was no choice. It would pass over less judgmental, less like she was desperate to escape back. "Umm, I've got other friends coming to visit soon. I need to get back." Reluctantly, Julie and her father began the long, awkward car Journey back to the hospital, where each minute felt like ten.

Back on the ward, Julie went to her room. She was dying to cut herself. She lay on her bed, looked at the time. She closed her eyes and imagined the quick sharp movements of cutting herself, of feeling the release as the blood flowed down her arm. How heavenly that would be. What a relief she would feel.

She must be an evil person for her sister and mother to hate her so much. There must surely be something evil about her, or why else would people hate her with such diligence? What was wrong with her? Why did they hate her so much? Was it justified? All these thoughts were racing through her mind, giving her a dizzy headache.

Death by psychiatric ward. I prefer death by chocolate.

Chapter 8

"It's too hard!" she sobbed to John on the phone, "it's just too hard. The pain is too much. It's all such a struggle. I just want to disappear..." loud gasping sounds were crying down the phone.

As usual, John remained his quiet, contained self. He did not yell at Julie, he did not cry at her. He kept his cool and calmly replied with, "I know it may feel like that now, but it will get better. You just got to keep believing it, and trying. I think you can do it." His little words of encouragement were said so matter of fact, erupting with kindness and compassion. John truly, completely cared about her. He was giving her so much, and she was taking so much. He had spent over an hour on the phone to her each day, talking to her, showing such signs of selflessness. Julie was in love with him. She was not sure how she was in love with him, she just knew she was. He was safe, and he expected nothing back from Julie. He was beyond the call of human nature.

That was all said before he let her down. She asked him if she could come and stay with him at the weekend, a break from hospital, a relief. But no. He said no. He did not care. He was far too busy.

"I feel funny," Julie tried to explain to Sarah.
"What do you mean funny?"
"I don't know how to explain it. Someone is following me. Something evil is around..."
Sarah gave Julie a pen and paper. "If you can't explain it, try writing it down. Julie started writing:

I walk around in a paralysed glaze. I can feel my body is somewhere on the floor, but I am somewhere in the air. My chest has such a heavy, depressed feeling that I feel weighed down with the burden. I walk around. I know my feet are touching the floor, but I know that I am unaware of how or why I am moving.

It is then when I know they are there. The evil feelings are so strong they are being made into a person. It is a monster within the walls, taunting me. I am being followed and pursued by this evil presence. I can feel the cold hatred running through the walls as it runs through my veins. The presence is torturing me, screaming out so much evil I find it hard to resist screaming. I cover my ears, try to block out the sounds, but I can't. I run faster and faster to escape the sounds, but they travel like air. How dare you be ill. How dare you be alive. You should die. You should die. They are cursing me, controlling my mind. I am immobilised in their power. Kill yourself.

I am not real. I am not a real person. I am not supposed to be alive. I am wrong. It was a mistake that a person like me was born. I don't deserve to live. I should be punished. I need to cut myself to punish myself and make me feel calmer. What is wrong with me? Why do I feel like this?

Lauren was the ward brat, the pubescent adolescent. She liked to think herself as queen of the ward. She would strut around, shouting, kicking and swearing. When she walked in to a room, she expected people to either shudder in fear, or bow to her. She had bright ginger hair, and a face as pale as the cocaine she snorted when she had leave from hospital. If Julie had learnt anything, it was to avoid conversation with Lauren.

Lauren was in constant contact with Julie's sister. They texted, met up at the pub, encouraged the mutual hatred they had for Julie. She was the one who was bitching to Julie's sister, lighting a flame across an already flaky fire. Anything Julie said would be recorded, noted and reported back.

When Lauren was in a mood, everybody suffered.

"Fuck you; I want to get the FUCK OUT OF HERE. Fuck you fucking cunts. Get your fucking hands off me..." amidst these bursts of profuse anger, there were nurses pleading with her, trying to reason with her, calm her. These were not met with any form of human decency. They were met with violence and aggression, both verbally and physically.

Julie normally avoided Lauren at dinner, but it had been quite a few weeks now that Lauren had not shown her any hostility, Julie risked sitting there. What a mistake. Firstly, Lauren decided to show off that she had managed to have two vodkas in her coke bottle without any member of staff noticing. A conversation about benefits came up, and Julie admitted to receiving sixty pounds a week.

Lauren slammed her fork on the table. "Why the fuck do you get benefits? You used to be a teacher, you've shown you're capable of working? Why the fuck..."Julie continued putting mouthfuls of apple crumble into her mouth.

Eventually Julie wanted to shut her up, "it's none your business if I receive benefits!" Then Lauren got up and left.

A kind Patient with two plaits and a lot of makeup took Julie's side and empathised. "That girl, she's a bully. She targets people. I hate bullies."

Julie finished up and put her bowl in the bin, cautiously walking back to her room. But who should she bump into at the top of the stairs? Lauren was there, waiting for her.

"Don't you dare snap at me like that again."

Julie turned her head. "You started on me first. You're a bully." She was not going to let Lauren push her around.

Lauren pointed her finger in her face. "You're a stupid,

attention seeking little bitch who needs to get a grip."

Julie merely responded with, "alcoholic."

Lauren had her hands round Julie's throat. Julie was thrown against the wall. She pushed Lauren and ran crying to James.

"Lauren's trying to strangle me. She had her hands round my throat!"

James walked Julie to her bedroom. Gave her instructions to sit there whilst he dealt with Lauren. Julie waited. She burst into choking, vibrant tears. They were streaming down her face like waterfalls, and she could not stop them. James did not come back, she sat there, crying her sobs. Eventually she heard Lauren's voice, shouting she just hit me for no reason... and Julie waited to be told she was lying.

Sure enough, James came back and confessed that Lauren had given a very different account and that Julie had started it. It was a lie, an evil lie. James said he did not know who to believe and to keep away from Lauren. There was doubt in his voice. Julie felt isolated. She wanted to die now, really die and get away from this. There was far too much evil in the world. Julie did not want to be a part of it.

She was so angry. She could feel the boiling fur from the pit of her stomach and reaching out to her entire body. She sat on her bed, paralysed with anger that she could not control. This anger was a black force controlling her body. She wanted to cut herself. She closed her eyes and imagined cutting herself really deeply so that she could watch the blood oozing out of her arm. She looked at the time. She had to wait the twenty minutes. How could she wait twenty minutes? She was desperate to rid her body of the anguish she had just experienced, and the feeling that she was shunned into her room, hushed away. Prohibited. Julie was prohibited from the world.

Sarah was one of the nurses that spoke to Julie like she mattered. She came into her room and Julie felt that she cared. She sympathised with Julie, and it cheered her up slightly, but not enough.

"Is there anyone who can be with you tonight? Any friends?"

Julie phoned up Simon, her ex boyfriend Simon.

Simon and Julie had a complicated relationship. Much more complicated than her relationship with John. Whilst there were times when Julie and Simon argued profusely, there were also times of great love and connection. Despite their constant defensive bickering, they were both rather fond of each other in the end. They had to have one or two dramatic arguments before getting on with the day ahead.

Julie walked around the ward in a daze. She walked round the corridors. The blue unfriendly carpet felt rough under her feet. The white doors, with numbers being the only symbol to differentiate, greeted her coldly as she wondered. She listened to the evil inside the walls. Kill yourself. Die. Die. It would be better to be dead. You have nothing. Nobody would care. Kill yourself.

James was not working that night. Instead she decided to speak to Paul. Paul was tall and half Chinese, and these half features were present in his face. Not quite English, not quite Chinese. Just Paul. He was in the middle of giving out the tea time medication and stood behind the medicine counter which resembled a stable door, but instead of a horse peering out there was Paul handing you your pills. Julie stood at the door.

"I feel weird..."it was so hard to explain. How does one begin to describe the terror, the victimising of the evil voices shouting at you? How on Earth can Paul do anything to stop them?

"In what way weird?" Paul responded with the usual

concerned, but withdrawn manner.

"The voices are evil. They are telling me to die. They are scaring me I don't know what to do."

Paul raised his eyebrows in surprise, and looked down awkwardly at his hands. He seemed confused, yet saddened. He looked Julie straight into her eyes and said, quite simply, "well I don't want you to die."

Julie went to her room feeling calmed.

Chapter 9

Julie was growing tired of the hospital. It was never ending. At first she had felt relieved to be there, thankful that she could be safe from herself and her tortures, but now she wanted to leave. The walls were closing in on her, trapping her. She wanted to discuss these new thoughts with Doctor Slater. However, there was also something terrifying about the idea of leaving, something so scary and unforeseen Julie did not know how she would cope. She needed the hospital ward. She needed to be around people, to be allowed to be mentally ill if she was. She was stuck.

Ward round was the usual specimen experience. In a room full of doctors, therapists, pharmacists, nurses and social workers, Julie was the specimen they were all there to watch and to react to. A bear in a swarm of bees, a knitting needle amongst ordinary needles. Julie focused all her attention on Doctor Slater, and the rest all merged together just to form the background of ambiance.

On a piece of paper in front of her eyes, Julie had her points written down so that she would remember to discuss everything. How she was bored, felt like nothing was happening, that she was stuck in a hospital ward and felt like prisoners were treated better, for at least they knew when they would be released.

Doctor Slater began to ask her about medication, mood and the frequency of self-harm. Suddenly Julie's voice grew into a malicious lump that was wedged into her throat. Words escaped her, and her body felt numb. Her surroundings mingled into one swirl of unreal matter that could be called humans. She tried to speak, but no sound came out. She had known the doctor was talking to her, she knew her social worker was touching her hand, which she whisked away in confusion. She could not bear this; she could not understand what was happening. It was not until she got up and walked out the room that she started to feel again, but she was still numb. Walking on the air. She went back to her room and cut herself, and felt the very real sensation of warm, stinging blood trickle down her arm. She was human again, she was real. She could feel the pain.

The next day she decided to phone her social worker to find out what had been decided for her future. Her social worker was a tiny woman, with certain maternal qualities but on a professional level. Julie neither felt anguish for this character, nor any form of bond. She was just there.
"Yes, I thought perhaps you were disassociating yesterday. We discussed two things; firstly about you attending the day services they have at WATS. These are therapeutic classes they run. Secondly we talked about the possibility of you moving to a halfway house in Watford. You'll have nurses there still, but it will be in a house technically, you'd still be an inpatient. How do you feel about that?"
Still panicked about the idea of leaving hospital, she was torn by her boredom as well. Reluctantly, she agreed that they both sounded like a good idea. One tiny step out into the community. One step towards normality. What a long Journey it was.

John was growing to become Julie's rock, her means of survival. She phoned him several times a day, whether in a state of fear, of suicide to keep her in touch with reality. She threatened suicide, cried so many tears down the phone to him. She was petrified she had driven him away, pushed him too far. She had to phone back after her psychotic episode just for the reassurance he would still be her friend, still be there for her when she needed. He responded calmly, and quite unemotionally. He reassured her that he would still be her friend. He told her she did not need to die, she did not want to die, and it was just what she was feeling now. John was her state of support, but Julie knew she was becoming increasingly dependent on someone who had no romantic interest in her. However many times he reassured her that he would still be her friend, she was expecting him to cut her off any minute, just like her other friends had done. It happened sooner than she would have liked.

The boredom of the psychiatric ward beseeched her. She had been there so long, for about four months now. She had seen the fall of snow about three inches deep, and now she was noticing the changes into spring. The sun started shining, the days grew longer, and Julie's impatience heightened.

Kerry looked dirty. She was in her forties, but could easily be mistaken for fifty. Her blonde hair looked messy despite however many times she combed it. Her face was red and patchy no matter how many times she washed it. Julie saw her for an ugly person on the inside which was seeping through into her appearance. She had been friendly at first, greeting Julie and welcoming her on the ward. It did not take long for her true colours to leak through this image. She started swearing and growing more and more aggressive.

"My name's Kerry. Sorry about that," she started, slamming the living room door. "You can go fuck ya self an' all!"

One evening Julie was feeling fed up. She was bored of being ill. Hell, she was bored of being bored. She really fancied curling up in front of the television, or having a nice shower then cooking herself some pasta. The hospital could be suffocating.

"I wanna go home!" Julie whinged to Kerry on the

On a Knife's Edge

table.

Kerry stared down at the leek and potato mess on her plate. She put her fork down and pointed at Julie with her grubby fingers. When she spoke to revealed yellow, smoke stained teeth. "I have had just about enough of the likes of ya. You are such a spoiled ungrateful brat. You could go home any time you fucking want. The only reason you're fucking here is cos you take a fucking slice out of ya arm now and then. Fink you're fucking clever? Me, I gotta stay here. I got real problems, me darling. I ain't seen my kids for weeks. I am a fucking alcoholic and its way more serious than any silly problems you may have, you little cunt."

Julie had knots in her stomach. All of her body as wrenching to start crying, but she refused. She had to say something, something small, something to show Kerry she was not such a weak, pathetic little girl. With a tiny voice she simply murmured, "I'm glad I'm not you." Kerry started swearing away in response, but Julie ran away.

When she was safely hidden in her room, she locked the door and let the tears spill.

It was shortly after this incidence Kerry was beaten. Again, during a meal time, Kerry acted out. She started shouting at the nurses that she was human, and that the nurses were all cunts. One African nurse stood up to her. "Don't speak to me like that!"

Kerry grabbed her with her fists, shouting racist insults in her face. The nurse, with people's encouragement, called the police. The next day, one of the doctors made Kerry leave. Then once again, for a short time only, all was quiet on the Eastern front.

It was time for lunch, a time for the school bullies to come out to play. Julie, small and meek, dreaded this escapade. She was afraid to eat by herself, yet she was afraid to talk to anyone. She had a chicken tikka sandwich in her bag. She went up to the group of girls from another class sitting on the grass. The sun was shining down strong, and this was the spot for the sunbathers. Hoping they would just ignore her, Julie started eating her sandwich. No such luck.

"Ewww! What are you eating? That smells so bad!" Jennifer was the leader of the group, and quite possibly the ugliest girl Julie had ever seen. "What is it? Yuck, it stinks like shit."

Now the girls turned around and stared at Julie, grinning away. This was brilliant! Julie was so sad and uncool, and they were the cool ones picking on her. They started taunting her, making as many nasty comments as possible.

"You know, fat people should wear stripes going down. If you ever wear clothes with stripes going around your tummy, you'll look even fatter!"

"Oh my God! Look at her shoes! Julie your shoes look so sad. Why are you wearing them?"

"Ha ha! Ugly shoes with white socks. That's just wrong!"

It was one comment too many. Julie could not stand it. Her lower lip trembled as she fought back tears. She gathered up her things in such haste that she dropped a few books, which was met with a chorus of laughter. Julie felt like the village idiot. She hurried over to the maths block that stunk of dust because nobody ever hung out in there. She thrust open the heavy toilet doors, and let the tears spill over. She cried and cried until she had no tears left in her chest to shed.

He did not phone. He promised to phone in ten minutes but that was two hours ago. Where was he? Why didn't he phone her? Everybody lets you down. Nobody cares about you. The whole world is such a horrible, cruel place. It's a cruel world after all.

Chapter 10

Everyone had a charge nurse, the nurse that was supposed to speak to their Patients on a daily basis. James was Julie's nurse. He was tall and lanky, with white hair and deep blue eyes. On first meeting, he had such an air of compassion that Julie felt instantly at ease. Like a lot of Julie's relationships, she began by greatly admiring Justin, and ended up hating him. However, as promised, he sat down to talk with her.

She started to unburden all her frustrations of the hospital ward. The nurses' reactions to her self-harm, the nurses' comments, the other Patients and how they were all forced to suddenly live and spend time with strangers. She was starting to hate hospital. She was starting to hate herself for feeling so depressed and not seeming to be able to do anything to feel better. What was wrong with her, why did she feel so bad? Sometimes they said there must be a reason. But there was no reason. She just was depressed. It's obviously something wrong in your brain, John told her. Something deep and biologically complicated. Give it time. Time; time was all she had.

James tilted his head in empathy. "You know, I can tell from your posture that you are feeling depressed. I sense it in your figure. But, Julie, it always seems to be the same thing. There always seems to be this conflict about how the nurses treat you. What can we do to make this better?"

Julie sat silently. She hated the medical staff asking her questions she found challenging to answer. She looked at her feet and started gently swinging them back and forth childishly in her chair. For some reason, she felt like bursting into tears.

"I want to train the nurses. I have already been a teacher before. I want to be able to train nurses how to act around the Patients, to stop them saying silly, ignorant things. How can I do that?"

"I have a number here for a Laura Ballen. She works with service users. Why don't you give her a call and see if you can contribute anything?"

"Um, yeah ok. Maybe I'll give that a try..."

After speaking to Laura, Julie was invited to become part of an interviewing panel for a head of psychiatric nurse for the new psychiatric hospital in Harperbury. She was actually going to assist in the recruiting. She was actually going to have a say in what type of person will be looking after others like herself. She may eventually have some value in this world.

Form time in year seven was the worst out of all her school years. It was that dreaded twenty five minutes between taking the register, and waiting for the bell to ring for the first class. Those twenty minutes were pure torture for Julie. She felt the familiar pang as once again, she was sitting on her own on the front bench. A purple rucksack in front of her, with straps so played with they were permanently crooked. All around her, children were laughing, joking and bantering. But not Julie. She was by herself, away from the class.

When nobody spoke to Julie for most of the day, she used to pinch herself to make sure she was still real. People in her class form did not know she was real, but being invisible was preferable to the verbal abuse she regularly had to face. She longed so much to be a part of a group, to be meaningful, but she was nothing. She was not wanted on this planet.

Not only did she have to put up with this anonymous torture in the mornings, but the devil himself arranged for more form time in the afternoons. Granted, it was slightly shorter than morning registration, but it equally played a means of suffering for Julie. She was

On a Knife's Edge

subjected to evil comments, most commonly were "loner," "sad," and "fat". Julie grew to despise herself, particularly the way she looked. She had a pretty face, but her body was rather plump. She absolutely hated herself. She started to pinch herself more often, just to punish herself for being so fat and repulsive.

The pinching made her feel real. It was her only friend and she remained under total control. One morning, Mr Wilkinson came in late, and accidently knocked his coffee mug on the floor and it shattered in pieces. Julie, pleased for something to distract the nothingness, jumped up and started to help him. She picked up a sharp piece of china, and looked at it lying in the palm of her hands. She looked around at the others, all sitting up at the ugly wooden science lab tables. They looked happy, cheerful, and oblivious. Yes, Julie had a secret that they did not know, as they did not know she had some china in her hands. Without thinking too much about her actions, eleven year old Julie squeezed that sharp china in her fingers, and watched the blood trickle down her hands to stain her blazer.

Julie was greeted with just as much isolation when she returned home from school. In her mother's eyes, Julie was tough and independent, whilst her little sister Jenna was in much more need of her mother's nurture. Jenna was extraverted and would cry and scream until she got her way. Julie's mother and Jenna would lock themselves up in the living room, constantly crying and supporting each other. Neglected, Julie sat in front of the television sometimes, but often she would go to imagination land.
In imagination land, Julie was adopted. Her real mother was a beautiful, thin and elegant woman with long, flowing blonde hair. She would ride a horse through the fields of Bushey leading into her back

garden. She would stop at their fence and beckon for Julie to come down to greet her. Then she would scoop Julie up in her arms, and ride away with her.

The thing Julie needed most in the whole world was a mother. A mother to love her. That was when she met Emma.

Julie watched the rain fall from inside her hospital room. The rain was pouring down hard. She was supposed to be going to her psychologist this morning. She could feel the tension rising in her stomach at the thought. She would have to rush to her appointment in the rain, then rush back to the hospital for an appointment with the doctor, her social worker and John was even coming as the social worker told her she could bring someone to the meeting for support.

The psychologist was due to see her at half past nine. The doctor was due to see her at half past ten. This meant she would have to be sure to leave the doctor by ten fifteen, ultimately skipping the last five minutes. It would be a forty five minute meeting as opposed to a fifty minute one. No problem. What was five minutes?

Stressed, Julie dashed over to Upton Road. The rain was getting heavy. She could feel the water soaking up her jeans, splashing her legs. She was drenched by the time she reached Upton Road. Her hair hung straggly by her shoulders. She was out of breath from power walking to reach her appointment. It was really important she was not late as it would already have to be cut short.

After announcing her arrival, Julie sat in the waiting room drying off and waited for Alex. She was conscious that is was now twenty five to ten. Five minutes now lost. Still nothing. She began to grow very uneasy. Where was he? Where the fuck was he?

At twenty to ten, she got up and asked the receptionist.

On a Knife's Edge

She simply shrugged her shoulders, mumbling something about he must be running late. Julie could do nothing but sit and wait. She could not concentrate on her book. She picked up a magazine and started flipping through, but in the end gave up and started playing Sudoku on her phone. By a quarter to ten, Julie was almost in tears. She could feel the overwhelming feelings of anger and panic wedged deep within.

When Alex finally arrived, Julie had shut herself off from the world. She was so cross, she could not contain it. She could not simply put on her happy mask and continue. No, she was furious. Alex immediately picked up on this, and was instantly in tune to how angry she was about her time being cut so short. He started to ask Julie questions. She looked at him. Oh, how desperate she was to answer him. How she tried to listen and respond, but something in her body shut down. She was unable to talk, unable to engage in conversation. She lost the will to live right before his eyes.

As there was clearly no point in continuing, Alex ended the session fifteen minutes early.

Back at the hospital, John was waiting for her. He was standing in the rain, a folder over his head in a rather amble way to protect him from getting his hair wet, but failing. He towered above Julie, and his work clothes made it look like he could have been a consultant. For some unknown reason, Julie was intimidated by John's presence.

John and Julie waited impatiently outside the art room for the psychiatrist to summon them in. After about half an hour and three cups of decaffeinated coffee later, they were called in. Julie sat beside Pauline, her social worker with her back rest to prevent her slipping. John took the only available seat, right next to the consultant,

Dr Smith. As usual, he began with the introductions.

"Hello Julie. You know Dr Graham, Dr Frank, Mr Loory the pharmacist, Mr Woo the therapist, Mr Ben the bed manager and of course you know Pauline." Julie nodded.

"So, tell me Julie, how are you?" This question was impossible. Julie did not know how she was. Crap sometimes, fine the next. What a jumble of mixed emotions this question caused and Julie could only say in a tiny voice, "ok."

Dr Smith continued the familiar protocol. "So, how has your cutting been? Can I see your chart? Good, you've been sticking to the fifteen minutes. Do you think we can increase that to twenty minutes? Mr Ben, just to fill you in, Julie has a self harm log. She waits fifteen minutes after she gets the urge to self harm, and records it in her log." Mr Ben nodded. John peered over to try and see.

Julie was looking very worried. Twenty minutes? Why did he keep increasing it? This was pure torture. Nervously, she nodded her head. What else could she do?

"Now, Julie, we have plans for you to be moving off the ward shortly. You can go to a halfway house, based in St Albans. That way you can attend day services in St Albans town centre. You will not be able to attend the services in Watford because your sister is here. Do you understand what I am saying to you?" Julie was silent. "What I am saying is that you will still be an inpatient and you will still have to come and see me every week, but for the moment you are now well enough to go to the halfway house."

Julie was choked up with tears. She was so desperate to leave but at the same time she was terrified. How can she be so desperate to leave but so scared at the same time? The world made little sense.

Julie was upset. She was panicky. She did not know

why, but all she could feel were strong impulses to die. Strong impulses to put her handbag around her neck and strangle and squeeze and squeeze. No more pain, no more life. She felt desperate, so she went to find James, the charge nurse. He promised to come and find her.

Two hours later, no sign of James and Julie's depression was increasing. She went back to the staffroom, and James was on the computer. She asked again if he could speak to her.

"To be honest, Julie, you'll be moving to the halfway house soon. You can talk to them."

Julie felt a kick in the gut at this comment. "What? That's it? I'm not your problem anymore?"

James looked down at his oversized feet. "Actually no, Julie, you're not." Then he walked away, leaving Julie alone in the staffroom, paper blowing at her feet.

What James did not know was that Julie knew his secret. Sandra was a nice nurse, but her intelligence level was low. She was beautiful, a forty five year old Pilipino woman who could have passed for thirty. Her tiny waist went well with her big brown eyes. Sandra fell in love with Julie, consequently forgetting the necessary professionalism between Patient and staff. Sandra spent time with Julie like two teenage girls at a sleepover.

"Hello, darling. Let me do you make up, yes?" Sandra sat on the edge of Julie's bed, splashing make up on her face. "Darling, you so pretty. Your eyes are beautiful." She put her arm around her and gave her little kisses.

One evening Julie was completing a rather tedious puzzle of a random pond that looked quaint, when Sandra sat beside her and confessed that she was having a secret love affair with a married man.

Julie responded unenthusiastically, and slightly

disgusted, until Sandra showed her a picture of her secret love. It was James. Julie immediately jumped to attention. "Oh my goodness, that's James! Oh my goodness you're having an affair with James!"

Sandra giggled, then looked sad. "He doesn't treat me well. I know he doesn't treat me well, but I keep going back to him. I just love the sex."

Julie gasped in surprise. She could not believe her ears! "Yes, darling, I love the sex. James is so good at it it's so much fun. Yesterday we went to a hotel and did it all day. My legs are hurting so much today. But you cannot tell anyone, ok, sweetie?" Julie nodded obediently. Next time James was around she would have to observe his behaviour towards Sandra, catching any confirmations of flirting. James had two young children. She could not believe his behaviour.

Sandra continued her conversation by off loading onto Julie, telling her how she had to have an abortion due to James and how that had made her really depressed. Julie felt like the roles were reversed. She was now the nurse, Sandra the Patient.

She decided to give it a go. Yes, she would cry and show her mother how distraught she was. Maybe, just maybe, she would comfort her for a change. She cried out in sobs, "I miss Emma." Her mother started crying too, and Julie felt the anger rising in her throat. "Mum, why are YOU crying?"
Her mother started her crocodile tears, "because I miss Emma."

Julie vowed never to show emotion to her mother again. And she never did.

Chapter 11

Julie was in her room. She was terrified. There was a conspiracy going on, and she knew it. She was out to get her. Jenna was an ever present thought in her mind. Then she knew. Jenna absolutely despised her; that she was certain of. Her parents frequently reminded her about how much she was hated. So now it was obvious what was happening. Jenna was conspiring with the greater force to make Julie feel bad. Jenna wanted to control Julie's mind in order for Julie to kill herself.

The dark evil forces were seeping through the walls. The black feelings were surrounding Julie, capturing her. Jenna was a powerful person and she knew exactly what she was doing. Julie put her head in her hands and cried, begged for Jenna to leave her alone. The voices continued, whispering and willowing around her mind. Julie's screams were not loud enough to stop them.

In desperation to control the commotion in her head, Julie broke her razor blade off and cut herself repeatedly until all was calm and tranquil once again.

"A Pseudo hallucination?" Julie repeated.

"When you thought your sister was trying to kill you, was it in your head or in the room?"

"In the room. She sent black feelings to try and make me kill myself."

"Right, but they were in the room. Were they in a particular place or were they coming from all directions?"

Julie was getting discomforted. Saying it now to doctor Salter sounded ridiculous, and she was very aware of that. "It was coming from all directions..." she said in a tiny voice.

"Right, ok so then it was a pseudo hallucination. Ok,

Julie, off you go."

Julie remained stuck to her chair. Her head started to swift and race away from her body. She found herself unable to respond to the doctor properly. Doctor Smith looked at her with some interest. "Julie, what are you thinking now?"

Julie did not know. She looked at the trees moving back and forth in the wind and thought of her friend Emma. "There's someone in the trees..."

"Look, Julie, try to think rationally. There is nobody in the trees. Try to be a bit more normal. Would you like some quetiapine?"

Julie shook her head. "No, thanks."

"Well, Julie, I think some quetiapine would be a good idea. I'll get the nurse to get you some, ok?" Julie nodded in agreement. Who can argue with the lord itself?

Julie was sitting in her room, staring at the peach colour ceiling, wishing that some excitement might occur. As always, be careful what you wish for. Her mobile phone started to ring, and when Julie looked at the name, she saw "mum" was calling. That was odd. Her mother never called her. She nervously answered it.

"Hi, darling. Look, I am going to pop over to the hospital and find someone I can talk to and ask them how I can help you."

Mortified, Julie agreed and went in search of a nurse she could forewarn. Paul was in ward round, James was not in today. The only charge nurse was a kindly man called Amar, but Julie had never had much to do with this nurse. She told him her mother was on the prowl.

Her mother arrived with her usual clutter of handbags, carrier bags and baskets. She found Julie, and together they went in search of Amar. Good naturedly, Amar introduced himself, and then invited them both to sit in the staff room (where other members of staff would be in and out).

"So how may I help you?" Amar asked.

"I would like to see my daughter's notes please."

Amar shifted in his chair. "I'm afraid I can't do that. It is confidential."

"Well, I am her mother and I need to know how I can help her."

"Yes, but we cannot simply show you her notes. All is confidential; it is up to the doctor."

"But I need to see her notes. I need to know. Can you tell me a bit about her diagnosis and how I could help her?"

Before Amar could refuse again, Julie tried to rectify the situation. "No, mum, he's not allowed. But you can ask me. What do you want to know?"

Daggers shot through her mother's eyes. "No, I need to speak to a professional."

"Mum, he's not allowed to. Just ask me."

Amar suggested she wait to speak to the doctor. Furious, her mother responded that if Amar would not tell her anything, then the doctor would not either.

The throwing back and forth conversation went on for about twenty minutes, her mother asking questions, and Amar carefully not answering. In the end her mother gathered up her clutter and stormed out.

The next time Julie went round to her parent's house for dinner; her mother had something to say. "I need you to write a letter to your doctor, giving me permission to see your notes."

Julie placed the forks back in their drawer, now clean. "I don't think you can do that." What was she talking about? No way did she want her to see her notes.

"When I had breast cancer, you looked after me. Now it's my turn. You wouldn't have liked it if I hadn't told you."

In her head, Julie was screaming. I've been in that hospital nearly six months, and she has only come up to visit once. Once! She never phoned her daughter, never showed any indication that she cared, and now she wants to see her notes? Well, Julie was not going to write a letter, no matter how snappy and unpleasant her mother would now be towards her.

It was Christmas 1997. A fourteen year old Julie was sitting at the table, eating carrots. Shamefully, she also ate a bit of turkey breast, some roast potatoes and some stuffing. Oh my goodness. Why did I eat that? I can't believe I ate that. You are so fat and disgusting. It is wrong for me to eat. I need to get rid of it. I can't have it in my stomach it needs to go.
I got to go to the toilet and stick my fingers down my throat. No, it's not working. I need it to come out. I need to make myself sick I can't have the food inside me anymore. It needs to go. I am suddenly really really sick and I breathe a sigh of relief as the food comes out.
But it hurts so much. My stomach is crying out in pain. My mouth it sore and acidic, but at least the food is gone. The food is all gone.

A few months later, her mother and grandmother are talking.
"She needs a psychiatrist," insisted my grandmother, "she has anorexia or bulimia. She needs help."
"No, no, no, a psychiatrist is just going to blame it all on me and say what a terrible mother I am. She can't go." My mother is just as adamant.
But my grandmother stands firm. "No, you need to take her to one. She needs to go."

Each night I feel the same panic, the same fear and desperation. You should not eat, you don't deserve to eat, you are evil for eating. Each night I am on the

On a Knife's Edge

phone to Emma, crying, pleading with her. "Emma, I've eaten too much." Emma always said the same comforting thing, "no, you haven't. It's ok, you haven't eaten too much." Each night Emma says this to me, repeatedly over and over again. Emma is my angel. Emma is my saviour.

A bag without a handle
The dark without a candle
Then there's me without my best friend,
Emma

Emma Dinata. 1983-2000

Julie started packing up her belongings for the half way house. How strange to finally be leaving the hospital ward. She had so many belongings that had emasculated in a gigantic heap of rubbish. There was paperwork, benefit letters, scribblings, Sudoku puzzles, vogue magazine and a big pile of paintings. She spent a long time collecting up her things as she was going to be collected between ten and eleven am.

By five to ten, she was sitting on her bed, ready. It got to ten, but still nothing. They are probably going to be late. How was she going to occupy her time without going crazy with nerves? Luckily, Curtis came and asked her if she wanted to go into the art room, an ideal distraction. She got out her watercolours, and sat and started to paint. She painted her comforting image. It was a beautiful sunset of colours on a beach. In the distance she painted some mountains with little houses featured in the distance. This was her happy place.

By twelve o'clock, there was still no sign of the halfway house. She started to feel slightly discouraged. If they really wanted her there, then surely they would have come? She looked at the calendar on her mobile, and worked out that she had been there for about eight months. Eight months! She thought back to the CAT team that told her she would only be in one or two nights. She remembered sitting in that room with Anna all those months ago. It seemed like a life time ago now. Yet she was still depressed. She was still cutting herself. But before she used to cut herself five times a day, perhaps now it was three times. There were even occasions when it was once a day. Was that better? Or was it just as bad?

Suddenly, a lady poked her head through her door. "Oh, hello there. Susan; pleased to meet you. Right, let's get all your stuff down here. Blimey, you got a lot of stuff! Look at all those shoes. Right, let's get moving."

It took several trips down to the car, and it seemed to feel like they were clearing out a room after somebody had died. The mournful, sad feeling enraptured her as she brought down her pictures, clay models and her bags. Once all was done, Susan asked her if she wanted to say good bye to anyone. She desperately went searching for Curtis. He put his arm half heartedly around her, claiming he could not technically do anything else. The charge nurse handed Susan a box of her medications and some bandages. They were ready to be on their way. A young girl who looked about fifteen was waiting in the car and introduced herself as Clare, a student nurse. Of course that meant she must be at least eighteen.

The house was just that; a house and no longer a hospital. There were six bedrooms and a living room. There was a tiny kitchen and a nice garden. Julie was left to sit and sort herself out. She sat down on the sofa. Nobody was around. In the hospital there were always nurses and Patients around, but here she seemed to be left to her own devices. She was irrelevant again, isolated in the big scary world.

She phoned John and cried a little to him on the phone, and felt a bit better. So she went back to the quiet living room and flicked through the television channels. She left it on a programme, but was not really listening to anything. A moment later, her social worker walked in. Julie felt grateful to see the slightly new and slightly familiar face.

Pauline sat down on the couch and looked at Julie. Julie said nothing; she felt overwhelmed. Pauline started talking, and she saw the figure's mouth moving, but unable to respond. She then went up into her room and fell asleep.

Julie was bored, so bored. Her social worker set up an appointment on the high street of St Albans. She was due to go to a drama class this morning. Bloody hell! She had been to one of these groups before, a music group. It was so boring! They had sat around, listening to CDs. Nobody was allowed to speak, and Julie had to spend an hour of her life listening to bad sixties pop music. What a dire waste of her time. Well, she would give the drama group a try and see if that might be better. At least they wouldn't be able to sit in silence.

She entered 32 St Peters Street and was early, so she went into the common room. There were a lot of people sitting there, but nobody was speaking. Julie had the urge to cry, for this room of people were so unresponsive and quiet. She felt numb and wanted to burst into song, just to lighten up their day.

Up in the drama room Stuart walked in. He was fat and jolly and friendly. Julie warmed to him instantly, in one sense relieved that someone with a bubbly personality was there, and on the other sense a little nervous of his loud and boisterous character. He asked her if she wanted to go to the park for a bit before class started.

He sat in a small garden filled with roses and tulips, and rolled up a cigarette of tobacco. He did not stop talking. He told Julie all about his childhood. Apparently he was raised by goblins in a sewer and his parents were relinquishing the information. He then went on to discuss all the types of drugs he uses, and how he has been in an acute unit for two years under section. A lot for Julie to take in. She imagined running away from this bizarre character, running away from him and finding a life she had before where such mental health Patients were not in this world. She was now a part of them. She was part of the craziness, but she liked it. She could be herself.

Why did people do it? Why do they let you down? You go out of your way to help them, and then they toss you aside like you don't matter. It is so cruel and so unfair. Why is the world like that? Why? Why did she have to be born into such a horrible, nasty, selfish universe? It just seemed unfair. She had tried so hard to be kind and considerate to her. Laura, the girl from Mind with the same diagnosis of Borderline Personality Disorder. Julie had made friends with her, supported her. Helped her write an email to her doctor complaining about the poor quality of care. But Laura could not do anything in return. Julie gave up on her group to help her out, but Laura called five minutes before to cancel. Again. Julie was simply not important enough for people to keep arrangements. What a waste. She might as well just die.

On a Knife's Edge

Chapter 11

The average day for someone with borderline personality disorder is one emotional upheaval after the next. Anything might push you over the edge; an insensitive comment, a nasty tone, a promise not kept. The difference between people is those who can handle such events, and those who cannot. Unfortunately for Julie, she was the sort who found these such emotions impossible to deal with.

She had phoned the halfway house to announce she was going to be home late, and as the staff leave at nine then could they leave her medication out for her. They said they would, but when Julie returned to her old fashioned single bedroom, there was no medication to be found.

Julie wailed. And cried. And hit herself. She called the number they left with her for emergencies, but they did not have a clue who or where she was. She cut herself. Then she put her handbag round her neck and twisted and twisted until she felt dizzy and light headed.

She admitted to this act the next day, so a meeting occurred. They decided that when it was possible, Julie would move to another place with twenty four hour care called Cordianhouse. It was at this place that began her second phase of illness.

Julie always remembered a quote from the lady at Mind. The first time you become ill you reach the lowest point. After that, whenever you become ill, you never go back to that point because somewhere along the way you have learnt something. You can never go back to rock bottom. The only other way is up.

www.ingramcontent.com/pod-product-compliance
Ingram Content Group UK Ltd.
Pitfield, Milton Keynes, MK11 3LW, UK
UKHW041413180426
11947UKWH00007B/99